10
NATURAL
REMEDIES
That Can Save Your Life

10 NATURAL REMEDIES

That Can Save Your Life

JAMES F. BALCH, M.D.

D O U B L E D A Y

New York   London   Toronto   Sydney   Auckland

This book contains information concerning some controversial and developing treatments. It is not intended as a substitute for the medical advice of your physician. The reader should regularly consult a physician in matters relating to his or her health, particularly before taking any medication or supplement, natural or otherwise, including in respect to any symptom which may require diagnosis or medical attention.

A MAIN STREET BOOK
PUBLISHED BY DOUBLEDAY
a division of Random House, Inc.
1540 Broadway, New York, New York 10036

MAIN STREET BOOKS, DOUBLEDAY, and the portrayal of a building with a tree are trademarks of Doubleday, a division of Random House, Inc.

10 Natural Remedies That Can Save Your Life was published in hardcover by Doubleday in 1999. The Main Street Books Edition is published by arrangement with Doubleday.

Book design by Lynne Amft

Library of Congress Cataloging-in-Publication Data

Balch, James F., 1933–
10 natural remedies that can save your life / James F. Balch.
p.   cm.
Originally published: New York: Doubleday, 1999.
Includes index.
1. Naturopathy—Popular works.   2. Alternative medicine—Popular works.
I. Title: Ten natural remedies that can save your life.   II. Title.
R733 .B253   2000
615.5—dc21   99-087660

ISBN 0-385-49350-9
Copyright © 1999 by James F. Balch, M.D.

Contents

Acknowledgments

THERE ARE MANY to whom I owe a great amount of gratitude and without whom this project would never have come to fruition:

My heartfelt thanks go to my beautiful wife, Dr. Robin Young-Balch, for her unwavering support and understanding. I thank my colleague, Ted Schwarz, for his endless hours of work and devotion; I thank my agent, Kevin, for being the liaison with Doubleday; my sincere thanks go to Jennifer Griffin and Patricia Mulcahy and numerous other people at Doubleday who have patiently assisted me throughout this project; I thank my legal right hand, Eva Martin; but most of all I thank you, dear reader, for caring about your health and the incredible value alternative health has to offer the quality of each of our lives.

10
NATURAL
REMEDIES

That Can Save Your Life

Introduction

I HAVE NEVER UNDERSTOOD the conflict between medical practitioners who seek natural remedies for their patients and members of the pharmaceutical industry. For thousands of years people of all nations and cultures have used the resources of the world around them in order to remain healthy. They gathered food from trees, bushes, and the ground, and combined exercise with wholesome foods. They paid attention to how they felt when they drank different teas made from the plants around them. They learned to hunt and then prepare the meat in ways that seemed to benefit them. And they sought fresh, unpolluted drinking water.

More active forms of health care were called on when people had accidents. The steps taken when a man was gored by an animal, broke a limb in a fall, was cut by rocks or tree branches, all led to what we know as surgery. In fact, most of the surgical procedures followed in the United States until approximately 1950, just a half century ago, were also performed in Rome in the first century A.D. The major difference between them was that the Romans had no knowledge of germs and antiseptic practices. The concept of antisepsis had to wait until Joseph Lister, in the nineteenth century. But complex surgery was carried out for close to eighteen hundred years with little change.

What was the result? People lived long, healthy lives. In

some cultures, like the Diné, whom we call the Navajo, death at an early age was considered a disgrace. Either the person who died or a family member had failed the Great Spirit and then performed no cleansing ceremony. A long, productive life was natural, and it was achieved without pharmaceuticals, health maintenance organizations, preferred provider organizations, or private insurance plans. Instead, the people of the past relied on the scientific application of natural remedies.

When I became a medical doctor, I took the Oath of Hippocrates. Many people think he was the first physician, which is far from the truth. That honor goes to an Egyptian who lived many centuries earlier, as far as we know. Hippocrates was actually the first diagnostician. He told people who were sick to lie outside, near the marketplace. They were to tell their symptoms to passersby, hoping that someone who had experienced the same problem would say what treatment had worked best for him or her. That treatment would then be written down so that all physicians and patients could share it. This led to the repeated use of effective treatments, and doctors were able to determine the approach they would use to restore a patient to health.

In this way, Hippocrates improved medical care by compiling a system of shared knowledge for the public good. He also laid down ethical boundaries for all physicians, limits not always recognized by today's makers of pharmaceuticals. Part of the oath is: "First, do no harm." And while pharmaceutical manufacturers are not in the business of hurting people, the ultimate test of every drug is the effect it has on the neediest of patients or on those in the most controlled environment. New vaccines tried without prior testing on members of the military led to Gulf War Syndrome, an incapacitating reaction to the protective injections given to service personnel before they departed for the Middle East. Antirejection drugs are tried on transplant patients immediately after surgery, even though complications may force a return to older, established drugs. The loss of human life is a factored risk with each new product; no one wants anyone to die, yet it is accepted that there will be some losses. This is not a consideration with natural remedies when used appropriately.

So-called primitive people learned in much the same way as Hippocrates. Native Americans observed that if they cut themselves and could not stop the bleeding, the application of spiderwebs quickly brought clotting. If they had headaches, tea made of willow bark eased the pain. These methods were scientific, even though the term was not used at the time and the validity of the science is rarely acknowledged today. Always, people have used observation, experimentation, and the analysis of gathered data to help one another.

It has been only in the last hundred years that scientists have begun seeking both an understanding and the control of their world. If willow bark tea eased pain, they wanted to know why. In learning the reason, they isolated salicylic acid, a variation of the ingredient found in aspirin, the most frequently used pain reliever in America. The clotting property of spiderwebs was isolated. Vitamins were discovered. Nutrients. Enzymes. Scientists studied the natural way to good health and identified the reasons that remedies worked. Then, once the first step had been taken in controlling the healing process, big business took over. Why not create, artificially, the properties found in nature, package them, and charge exorbitant sums for them? Why not mount a campaign to debase "folk remedies"? Why not subtly change the climate so that people will feel so dependent on pills and elixirs that they'll ignore what once assured them of natural good health? In fact, why not alter society in such a way that those who conform to the latest thinking will inherently lack good health? Then everyone will need pills. Everyone will pay huge sums of money for pharmaceuticals. Everyone will be more concerned about obtaining health-care benefits than about having satisfying work and a fulfilling home life.

Does this sound odd? This is just what has been done. For example, ill health at one time was limited almost exclusively to the rich. Certainly there were diseases that ravaged whole populations. The plague, carried by rats, spread throughout many areas with concentrations of people. Influenza caused widespread death in urban America into the 1930s. But for the most part, the common illnesses of today were once nearly the exclusive province of the rich. We know that among the most prevalent complaints in the United States today is depression. Much of the depression from which people suffer deeply enough to see their doctors is caused by three factors. One is the lack of full-spectrum light (daylight or the equivalent). The second is a sugar-rich diet. The third is the absence of one or more significant individuals with whom one can form a nurturing community.

The lack of full-spectrum light is almost omnipresent. In the past, people worked outside, in daylight, for a major portion of each day. Peasants and laborers worked on farms, tending livestock, constructing homes, digging roads. Shopkeepers, clerks, and businesspeople walked extensively or used horses, and the care of their animals required their being out and about during the daylight hours.

Only the rich stayed indoors. Women believed that their skin was loveliest when it was untouched by the rays of the sun. Their depression and dark mood swings were accepted as normal female characteristics. After all, women were the "weaker sex." And the healthy, robust, active, productive peasant women? They were different, an inferior breed.

This attitude even became the subject for humor, as seen in the following story, which made the rounds shortly after World War II, at a time when class consciousness was at its height. A man observed a child being carried every day to the expensive car of a wealthy matron. The chauffeur would place the child on the seat, drive him wherever he had to go, then pick him up and carry him inside. After watching this repeated regularly, over many days, the man approached the matron and asked, "Madam, can't your child walk?"

The woman turned with a haughty air and said, "Of course he can. But, thank God, he doesn't have to."

Funny? Not when you look at the statistics for death among wealthy males in this century. At one time, a fifty-year life span was not at all uncommon, and most causes of death involved obesity, lung cancer, and heart attacks; all problems caused by a sedentary life, smoking, and poor eating habits.

Another contributing factor to the poor health of the rich was the discovery and consumption of white bread. At the time white bread was invented, there was little to distinguish the rich from the poor, other than their grand castles and manor houses, their fine clothes, and their wealth. There were no cars to buy, no home theaters, no costly electronic toys for amusement. Consequently, the difference usually was a matter of sensual pleasures; from multiple wives to rare foods imported or prepared at great cost. And among these special foods served to royalty was the newly developed white bread.

White bread was—and is—extremely unhealthy, lacking many of the essential nutrients found in the dark whole wheat bread the peasants ate. It was also expensive, which, even though it lacked nutrition, made it a symbol: The rich were somehow better. Tragically, when the "little people" learned that the wealthy were eating white bread, they looked on their wholesome dark bread as a sign of their lower-class status. So, when the cost of making white bread came down, it became the bread of choice for everyone. White bread was the great social leveler.

Refined sugar moved into the diet of the wealthy in the same manner. There were numerous healthy natural sweeteners used by the peasants in different parts of the world; the sweetener might come from chopped carrots, from raisins, from a sweet fruit. Refined sugar was for the rich, but no one attributed to it the vast mood swings of their "betters." Now we know that a sugar-rich diet can cause depression, along with hypoglycemia and diabetes. Many "moody" people have found that simply eliminating most of the sugar from their diet brings them a feeling of true well-being.

Royalty relied on meat as the primary part of a meal; fruits and vegetables were secondary. The peasants, who could not afford meat and were not allowed to hunt on the estates of the wealthy, ate mostly fish and the fruit and vegetables they did not have to take to the marketplace. The result was that the wealthy, lacking the full range of nutrients needed to sustain good health, suffered from malnutrition. Even the idealized portraits of the Greek emperors on ancient coins show evidence of such problems as goiter.

The rich and powerful were not fools. They noticed that they were not as strong and alert and did not have as much stamina as the peasant class. But they justified this by looking on the poor as work animals. Peasants were to do physical labor. Peasants were to fight the wars. Peasants were another form of livestock, the physical similarities among all men and women, regardless of birth, being just coincidences. No farmer can pull a plow as well as a horse or an ox, yet no farmer thinks of himself as inferior to his livestock.

The third cause of depression is a more recent one. Humans were meant to live as part of a community. The first man, Adam, was unhappy until he had a close relationship with Eve. Studies of the elderly have found that retirees who live alone, whether because of widowhood or because they are "loners," die within three years of retirement. They develop depression and a loss of will to live after spending so many years in the community of their work. They may have hated their jobs and looked forward to retirement, but the forced social interaction of the workplace—whether on the assembly line or in the corporate boardroom—ensured an emotional stability that contributed to wellness.

Other studies show that the healthiest individuals are those who belong to religious organizations in which they participate, fraternal organizations, or athletic groups, like bowling leagues. Being married or living with another person reduces the severity of depression or eliminates it entirely. It is the psychological and emotional isolation from others that leads to severe depression and death.

But this third cause of depression is primarily a product of our times. It was not a problem of the past, as were the other two causes of depression in the rich.

Sadly, today we have learned how to level our differences. We all lead unhealthy lifestyles, styles unchallenged by the pharmaceutical companies that benefit from our foolish notions.

For example, take a look at the typical "health-conscious" office worker. First there is his work environment. We may joke about our cubicle existence, but those cubicles, lighted by tungsten or standard (limited-spectrum) fluorescent bulbs, are the norm for millions. Factories may seem to be vast open spaces, often with skylights, but they lack exposure to full daylight. Even those fortunate enough to sit by a window lose the benefits of daylight because it is diffused by the glass.

The exceptions are those rare workers who have replaced their fluorescents with full-spectrum lights. These specialty fluorescents, which provide the equivalent of natural daylight, are usually sold in plant nurseries because they're useful in the indoor growing of outdoor vegetation. They are also recommended for people with seasonal affect disorder (SAD). SAD sufferers generally live in regions of the country where winters have long nights and short spans of daylight. Banks of full-spectrum fluorescent lights can alleviate the depression caused by the lengthy darkness, yet SAD is an extreme version of what we all experience unless we make an effort to be in the daylight.

Adding to the depression caused by the lack of full-spectrum light in our cubicles or similar work environs is our use of computers for both business and recreation. Instead of going for a walk to relax, the typical American is likely to sit by the television set or spend time on the computer. What with using the Internet and playing electronic games, the new popular forms of "relaxation," we are contributing to our depression and anxiety.

Even portable technology has created problems. In a recent study by the University Neurology Clinic in Freiburg, Germany, cell phones were found to affect blood pressure. The study, published in the June 20, 1998, issue of the highly respected medical journal *Lancet*, showed that one's blood pressure rises from 5 to 10 millimeters when a cell phone is turned on. Consider that many of the people who use cell phones are in business or relationship circumstances that are highly stressful, and combine that psychological stress with the physical changes of the electromagnetic field of the cell phone: You have one more prescription for ill health. And this is compounded when the same people take pharmaceuticals instead of altering their lifestyle. The drugs have a biochemical stress factor that exacerbates the very problem they're supposed to correct. Another crisis created by our "advanced" civilization.

We delude ourselves about all this. We join health clubs in record numbers, and health club memberships are becoming an expected corporate benefit. As these are indoors, however, we deny ourselves the essential value derived from exercising in daylight.

Next, add the fact that new buildings, as well as many renovated buildings, are designed for energy efficiency, which often calls for sealed windows and inefficiently recycled air, air that may contain bacteria, spores, and allergens.

Then add the processed food, the high-fat convenience meals, and even the proliferation of such nonfoods as the artificial fat used in some new snack foods, and you have a recipe for illness. The more we seek convenience, the more we import our fruits and vegetables instead of obtaining them from our gardens or farmers' markets, the worse our standard of health. Home gardens and nearby farms allow us to obtain food that has not deteriorated during a prolonged shipping time. It will not have had preservatives added. And if we are careful, we can make certain the food is organically grown before we purchase it.

The "good life" we try to live menaces us with the hidden dangers of our conveniences. We are daily courting ill health.

Drinking water is another issue. There are problems nationwide, from contaminants leaching through the soil, pollutants illegally (and sometimes legally) dumped into waterways, and high mineral deposits like lime. Yet even the clean drinking water offered in our cities can be tainted. Major urban areas, like New York, use mostly copper pipes to deliver water from the treatment and filtration plants to residences. The water may pass all manner of tests for purity, but even the best water delivered through standard household plumbing can be a source of trouble. Why? Aging copper pipes release trace amounts of the mineral into the drinking water.

There is nothing inherently dangerous about copper—it is a mineral found in many multiple-vitamin tablets—but it is essential only in very small amounts. When your intake is increased by your consumption of the trace amounts in your drinking water, you may be ingesting enough to cause depression. In some cases, it could be that there is nothing wrong with you except excess copper, but your depression is severe enough for you to seek medical treatment. And what does the typical pharmaceutical-inspired physician do? Instead of asking for a detailed environmental description of your life, your water pipes, your exposure to daylight, and the like, he probably prescribes a mood-altering drug like Prozac. You may feel better with it, but unless you learn to examine your drinking water, your time spent in full-spectrum light, your working environment, and the makeup of the food you eat, the depression may be a chronic problem. You will view yourself as emotionally or physically ill, and that will add to your despondency.

WHAT'S WRONG WITH OUR PHYSICIANS?

It's the rare medical doctor who wants to hurt his patients, of course. We physicians have always wanted to give top-quality care to our patients. What we don't realize, however, is how much we are hindered by the pharmaceutical companies.

The manufacturers of drugs have long controlled the content of medical journals and the short courses often presented at conventions. The advertising fees these companies pay for the journal space ensure that the magazines survive. As a result, for many years the medical journals refused to carry articles dealing with alternatives to pharmaceuticals, especially nutritional supplements. That was why, when the inventor of Valium, at one time the most prescribed tranquilizer in America, found that the use of certain B-complex vitamins would afford the same benefit as Valium without risk of side effects or addiction, the story was buried in an obscure international journal with a circulation of perhaps five thousand. The major medical journals ignored the story because the parent company of Valium's manufacturer was a major advertiser in their publications.

Medical schools gain millions of dollars in research grants from pharmaceutical companies and little from either health food companies or what might be called agribusiness. They have no incentive to add nutrition courses to the medical school curriculum. In fact, medicine continues much as it did in the days when Hippocrates considered only ways to help the sick and injured. He did not look at ways to keep people healthy so they would not need a physician.

Medical doctors are a reactive force. Hospitals pay high salaries to emergency room personnel. They pay little or nothing to provide the community with the information and support needed to avoid the causes of ill health.

Medical schools rarely offer courses in preventive techniques. Hospitals and HMOs can be bureaucracies where everyone is expected to follow procedures that offer the least risk of lawsuits. This means providing basic checkups, dispensing medication, advising how to change your diet after the diagnosis of an illness, providing surgery, and the like. And insurance companies do not give money to hospitals for serving a community of people so healthy that there rarely are needs for physician services.

If you've ever seen or used the *Physician's Desk Reference* (PDR), the annual compilation of information about pharmaceuticals, you may not have realized that the information is provided by the manufacturers. This is information similar to informational leaflets required by the Food and Drug Administration (FDA) when the companies package their products for pharmacists. However, unlike the packaging for professionals, in any given edition of PDR, essential facts that can lead to misuse may be omitted or underplayed. This isn't the fault of the publisher or the compilers. It is the result of the manufacturers' control of which information about their products is made readily available.

Likewise, when doctors obtain drug samples from sales reps (detail men and women in industry jargon), they're being guided in the treatment of illness by people with a stake in the reliance on drugs.

Compounding the problem is that drug companies now advertise directly to consumers. National magazines, major newspapers, television, and radio run advertisements for medications for heart problems, arthritis, and other common problems. These advertisements tell you to request the product from your doctor. They steer your thinking and tell you what to demand. As a result, most doctors won't consider natural remedies, either because they don't know about them or because their patients insist on something else.

NATURAL REMEDIES

I'd like to say that there is a natural health answer that's perfect for everyone. I'd like to give you a formula for living your life in perfect wellness. Unfortunately, that's impossible.

If the work you love, the work that supports you and your family, involves long hours at the computer, it is obviously not realistic to think you can work outdoors. You could get a desk lamp with full-spectrum light, but most people don't do this. Instead, you'll probably deal with tungsten or regular fluorescent bulbs, taking control only when you're at home. (In fact, if you work at home, you could change all the lighting in your house.)

You can fix the healthiest of meals from the freshest produce available in your local supermarket, but even those foods have traveled long distances in supermarket trucks. Often, "fresh" fruits and vegetables have been out of the ground for three days or longer. Sometimes they've been treated with gas to force-ripen them, or coated with wax to make them look better, or altered slightly in some other way. No matter how much attention is given to the safety of treated fruit, studies by the University of Chicago and other institutions show that the longer the produce is out of the ground, the fewer the nutrients that remain in it. The food value of a tomato bought in a grocery store is far less than that of a tomato picked from your garden or a farm.

What is also frightening is that if you rely upon modern medicine to deal with problems of depression and stress, you may be creating a harmful situation. All pharmaceuticals pose risks to some people. A drug to which I may be so allergic that my consumption of it is life-threatening may be the one that's essential to your recovery from serious illness. Why? Maybe I react to the binder that holds the medicine together, and you don't. But neither of us will know until we take it—and then it may be too late for me, the one with the allergic reaction. I could become severely ill or crippled, or even die.

To make matters more difficult for the seeker of alternatives, the testing of natural remedies does not always yield accurate data. In modern pharmaceutical medicine, an antibiotic is added to a petri dish containing a quantity of bacteria. Then the bacteria are either killed or not. This may be an effective test for an antibiotic, but it tells us nothing about the far more complex chemistry within the body, the natural petri dish for testing remedies. Natural remedies are not magic potions that zap the "bad guys"; they become part of a potent biochemical reaction within the body, where they form antibiotic responses, strengthen the immune system, and alter the body in ways not possible for pharmaceuticals. But they do not work on their own, as pharmaceutical tests require of their products.

This is not to say that tests cannot be conducted, only that they are complex. For example, early studies suggest that some forms of rheumatoid arthritis can be successfully treated with a program of exercise, the use of heat to ease joint pain, and a diet that includes B-complex vitamins. But none of these, tested alone, would show a beneficial effect. When they are applied together, however, they change the body's chemistry, and blood tests carried out over time prove their efficacy.

Fortunately, the potential of natural medicine is becoming more widely understood and accepted. Medical doctors like me, nutritionists, biologists, and other scientists no longer view nonpharmaceutical remedies as either outdated or suspect.

Instead, a growing number of physicians, horrified by pharmaceutical side effects, dangerous drug interactions, and allergic reactions, are once again calling on natural remedies. They use contemporary scientific research to learn which properties of the various remedies are likely to work for their patient. They analyze a patient's lifestyle to see whether a slight modification may bring about a major transformation in health. And they improve the quality of the patient's life.

While I was preparing this book, I concentrated on the health concerns of a majority of Americans and assessed the natural remedies they can utilize to make drastic positive changes in their health. And when I finished my work, I realized that there are ten natural remedies that can literally save your life. They affect your cardiovascular system, your hormonal balance, your immune system, your lymphatic system, and the rest of your body. They have all been scientifically tested and are well understood by the medical community. They have no side effects, which means that you will not suffer the curse of pharmaceuticals—iatrogenic illness (illness caused by the doctor or the treatment).

If you are concerned about acting as your own doctor by adopting some of the suggestions in this book, please discuss the material with your personal physician. Your physician may be familiar with some of the natural remedies discussed and will be pleased that you are interested in this extremely safe alternative to many pharmaceuticals. If not, he or she will be able to determine that what is discussed will not create a problem for you. No matter what, both of you may discover a safe and proven way to ensure that you enjoy a quality of life that would otherwise not have been possible.

Chapter One

LISTENING
TO YOUR BODY

BEFORE WE LOOK AT the ten natural remedies that can save your life, it's important for you to have a basic understanding of your health. For although I'm a doctor, trained in biology, anatomy, biochemistry, and related sciences; although I went to graduate school and have continued to take specialized courses as part of my continuing training; although I read medical journals by the dozens and know scientific terminology that few people can pronounce and even fewer define; still, when it comes to your body, I don't know nearly as much as you do. No doctor does.

You know more about your body than your primary care physician, your health maintenance organization, your preferred provider, your medical insurance company claims reviewer, or anyone else. You've been sensitive to the subtleties of your health and feelings since birth, a reality no one else can match.

Remember when you were very little and constantly experimented with everything around you? You'd touch this, look at that, taste something else, just to see what it was like. You used your senses to explore the world around you, to learn about hot and cold, pleasant aromas and foul odors, what causes pleasure and what causes pain. You learned about bladder and bowel control. You learned about hunger, thirst, and exhaustion. You learned what it means to feel good, and you learned what it means to feel sick. Daily life was a series of scientific experiments to teach you to know yourself and your relationship with the world around you.

Not that any parent looked at this natural learning process as being essential for your adult years. Your parents, like most adults, probably got mad at you for getting dirty.

"Don't put that in your mouth!" they'd yell. "It's yucky!"

"Don't touch that! It'll give you an *ow*."

In this way they helped teach you cause and effect, as well as simple remedies for whatever troubled you, though, again, they were unaware of doing so.

"If you're so tired that you can't keep your eyes open, go to bed!"

"Take a hot bath to relax; you'll feel better."

"Of course you feel terrible. You've been out in the sun too long without a hat. Get a glass of cold water and go sit in the shade for a while."

"How can you be tired when you've been sitting around all day? Go outside and play. You'll have more energy."

"Drink your milk. You need it for your bones to grow. You want to be strong, don't you?"

Now you're an adult, and although you know a great deal about your health, you may not realize that you do. You no longer live with your parents, but you've probably replaced Mom and Dad with other authority figures. But remember, your parents always had your best interests at heart, and the new authorities—pharmaceutical companies, advertising agencies, even the business aspects of medicine—are concentrating on their own interests.

The medical business establishment, composed of pill makers, pill pushers, and men and women whose jobs exist only because you seek their care, do not profit from your being well. Not that all of them think this way; the establishment does include many caring, dedicated health professionals. It's the businesspeople, the ones who study the profit-and-loss sheets, who know they'll be looking for work if you're in good health. These profit-oriented people want to encourage you to mask your symptoms, to resist healing, to substitute drugs for wellness. If you take a pill to fight depression and it makes you feel better, you'll take more pills in the weeks and months to come. If, however, you stop feeling depressed without having had medication, neither the pharmaceutical companies nor the medical practitioners will get a penny of your money. This is why I ask you now, even before you read about the natural remedies, to return to the awareness of your body you had when you were a child.

STEP 1: HOW DO YOU FEEL?

If you were to ask medical professionals to specify the complaint they hear most often, they'd likely tell you that their patients are always tired. "I don't have the energy I used to," some will say. "I'm tired all the time. I drag myself out of bed on Monday morning, drag myself through the week, and no matter how I try to relax over the weekend, I go back to work on Monday feeling no better than before."

Other problems are mood swings, especially among

women, and frequent minor ailments—a cold, flu, an intestinal virus, and the like. It is as though you're never completely well. Each time you get over one problem, another pops up.

What you usually do not discuss with your physician is your lack of such complaints. For example, suppose you've been dragging about the office all morning, not being very effective. Because you don't feel all that great, you really don't want much lunch. But when you see that it's a beautiful day, with the sun shining, you decide to go for a walk; perhaps you buy a sandwich and sit outside to eat it.

By the time you return to the office, you're surprisingly refreshed. You find yourself more productive; you're handling tasks that seemed impossible that morning; you're accomplishing work with more speed than you expected.

Perhaps you experience something similar on what you expected to be a bad day. It's raining, and you can't find a decent parking place. You have to park several blocks from work, and walk briskly to get to your office on time. You may be wet and cold by the time you arrive, but you feel elated somehow.

You also may feel better after interacting with another human being. You go to your church, synagogue, or mosque for the spiritual uplift it offers you. But have you noticed that the greatest joy comes after the service, when you're talking with others in the adult Sunday school or during coffee hour? It's the chance to talk, to share, to be involved with different people that uplifts you.

It's like that, too, when you're playing with your children, enjoying a pet, or spending intimate time with a lover. These experiences bring you pleasure. But you probably don't make note of them, the way you'd remember a pain, because doctors don't ask you about such experiences. In the past you were always taught to focus on negative things, not positive ones.

The good news is that when you focus on *all* your feelings, when you think clearly about what happened before, during, and after your experience, you're acting as your own physician. You're discovering what makes your body feel good or bad. You are discovering what has a positive effect on you and what has a negative effect. And when you're honest about these feelings and events, you'll have more knowledge about your health than the best doctors can acquire.

Note: It's important to separate natural good feelings from those that come with the use of recreational drugs—like nicotine, cocaine, alcohol, or even the heavy use of caffeine. Many people resort to recreational drugs because they give instant pleasure. They may be stimulants or depressants. They may briefly improve your ability to think, the way that drinking coffee does when you're working at your desk. Or they may make you feel that they're boosting your energy and mood, the way cocaine and nicotine do. But artificial stimulation always has a downside. Even if you set aside health issues and, in some cases, legal questions, you'll find that the most negative aspect of such artificial mood alterers is that they put your body on a roller-coaster ride. You may go up for a while, but you always go down—and you usually go down hard. The brief stimulation of the coffee may be followed by a period of greater tiredness. The high of coke or similar drugs may be followed by depression and a craving for more of the stimulant, enough that, for the heavy user, it becomes all-consuming. This is why such stimulants are ineffective at best, dangerous at worst. And this is why they have no place in your life or in your analysis of your health and your feelings.

Most doctors are trained to react to your symptoms by seeking the immediate cause but not necessarily the underlying cause. An illness, theoretically the problem, may actually be the symptom of something deeper, something wrong with your lifestyle.

Suppose you have an infection, the doctor prescribes an antibiotic, and you get better. Then, after a couple of weeks, you get another infection. Again, you're given the antibiotic. The cycle repeats itself. Throughout, the doctor continues to treat you in the same way. A quick glance at your records elicits a compassionate comment like, "You certainly have had a difficult year this year with all those infections." He gives another, stronger prescription for you to take to the pharmacist. And you, not knowing better, mumble thanks for the physician's concern, certain that he's done the best that can be done.

An antibiotic may help to fight each infection, but it does nothing to prevent the next one. Also, a common side effect of most drugs is a worsening of symptoms the next time you get the infection. This is because traditionally, doctors have been trained to treat symptoms, not the basic problem. And this is why your doctor usually will not try to determine why your immune system is unable to fight the infection that keeps repeating itself. This is why you, the expert on your own body, must look beneath the symptoms to find the lifestyle choices that may be causing them.

POP QUIZ

On a sheet of paper, answer the following questions.
1.   Do you go outside for exercise of any sort, including a brisk walk, at least twenty minutes a day, every day? Do

you do this during the daylight hours, regardless of the weather?

2. Is your lighting delivered by standard fluorescent bulbs? Incandescent lamps? Full-spectrum fluorescents?

3. Do you eat fast foods, fried foods, or foods with high sugar content three to five times a week or more? (Keep in mind that most commercial cereals, as well as pastries, doughnuts, and the like, fall into this category.)

4. Do you eat sweets as snacks, dessert, or with some frequency?

5. Do you find that caffeine doesn't affect you very much? Have you noticed that, even if it gives you a lift in the morning and midafternoon, it doesn't interfere with your ability to sleep?

6. Do you drink tap water? If you do, whether at home or on the job, does it come through pipes made of copper?

7. Do you drink water to quench your thirst, or do you get your liquid from juice, tea, coffee, and sodas?

8. Do you engage in a social activity like bowling, participate in a religious group, play on a sports team, attend club meetings?

9. Do you have a committed relationship with another person? If not, are you seeking one, or are you enjoying the casual style of "playing the field"?

10. Do you travel much by air?

11. Do you travel in a way that requires you to change one or more time zones?

12. Do you use a computer at work? At home? Both?

13. Do you relax with television or a computer?

14. Does your work schedule require you to commute before the sun is fully up or after it has set?

15. Are your work hours irregular, perhaps the first shift one week and the third shift another?

16. When you work the third shift, do you come home when others are waking up and getting ready to go to work?

17. Do you smoke?

18. Do you live with a smoker or work where you're exposed to cigarette, pipe, or cigar smoke?

19. Do you take any form of nutritional supplement?

20. Do you cook for yourself or rely on packaged foods that need only to be heated?

21. Do you eat beef? Pork? Chicken? Turkey? Fish?

22. Are you a vegetarian? Do you rely on a variety of vegetarian sources to give yourself the full range of protein your body needs?

23. Do you work or live in a building that recirculates the air, or do you have a constant source of fresh air, like through open windows?

24. Are you able to sleep through the night, or are you interrupted by small children, a sick family member, or someone else?

25. Do you drink alcoholic beverages or regular soft drinks?

Those twenty-five questions in Step 2 do not have right or wrong answers. Nor are they meant to serve as a guideline for a series of changes you must make. Rather, they're the questions that your physician should ask you when you have a physical exam. The answers may be significant indicators not only of your health but of the reasons you feel the way you do.

In most instances, working within your lifestyle to make the changes in habits with known negative health consequences will restore you to full wellness.

For example, high-sugar foods, beverages containing caffeine, many fried foods, and cigarettes are all factors in hypoglycemia—low blood sugar. Although they may bring a brief spurt of energy—you think clearly and are eager to tackle office concerns, chores, or active play—the rush of sugar to the body is followed by a shot of insulin needed to process the sugar, a shot as large as the one needed after a big meal. (The body starts to metabolize a candy bar, for example, with as much enthusiasm as it needs to tackle a four-course meal.) So after the sugar has been handled, you're suddenly in great need of something to keep the energy flowing. Unlike a healthy meal, which releases natural sugars over a matter of hours, keeping you active and alert from meal to meal, these sugar- and caffeine-rich foods send your body soaring up and plunging down. You rapidly rise to a peak, then crash, and you become so sleepy that you can't think clearly.

Before there's long-term damage, you may find yourself dozing at your desk, lacking the required alertness on an assembly line, fighting for control of your car, or in some other way being dangerously ineffective. Ultimately your immune system becomes weakened. You catch a cold, and just when you're getting over it, you're bothered by the sore throat and runny nose of yet another infection. Determined to work, though, you go to the office, where you drink coffee to stay awake, grab a doughnut or candy bar to give you energy at midday, and often bring fast foods to your desk for lunch because you have work to complete and may have to go home early to fall into bed.

Your exercising peters out. You may try to work out at a health club or gym, if that's been your routine, but you find yourself dragging. You certainly aren't going to do much walking outside, especially if the weather's bad. As a result, your exposure to daylight drops dramatically, and the immediate consequence is greater damage to your immune system, accompanied by a deeper depression.

The seriousness of this situation was described by researchers at Johns Hopkins University Medical School in Baltimore. Daniel E. Ford, the lead author of the article, reported in the July 1998 issue of the *Archives of Internal Medicine* that studies done over a long period of time show an increased risk of heart attack in men who suffer from depression. At this writing it is not certain whether the risk is associated with the antidepression medication the men took or from the physiological damage related to the depression.

When you describe your symptoms to your doctor, he or she will probably prescribe an antibiotic or some other pharmaceutical for the low-level infections that keep plaguing you. Maybe an antidepressant or a mild stimulant. In some instances, when the pattern continues, the doctor may make a diagnosis of chronic fatigue syndrome. Each day becomes a struggle, and you're thankful that the medications are keeping you from feeling worse. What you don't realize is that the lifestyle issues pinpointed by the quiz are the actual causes of your problem *and* the key to recovery. And you don't query your physician, because she's doing the job you expect. Unfortunately, wellness demands you to expect much more. It requires you to take charge of your health and use the knowledge you'll acquire in this book to adjust melatonin, antioxidants, diet, and other factors that may stop the problem, not just the symptoms, which is what medicine does.

Ironically, the reason that your physician may overlook the true causes of your complaints is that medical care has improved. In recent years we've garnered more knowledge about human physiology, anatomy, and biochemistry than we ever had before. We can do brain mapping, genetic analysis, and DNA plotting. We not only can perform surgery on organs whose damage once led to permanent disability or death, but we can replace organs. Liver transplants, heart transplants, kidney transplants, and numerous other complicated procedures are now so routine that there's an expectation of long-term success. In fact, many of the liver-transplant patients of just a few years ago no longer will need to take years of antirejection medication, because their bodies have already adapted to the foreign organ.

So what's wrong with contemporary medicine? It's become too technical, too specialized, and too narrow to ensure the wellness of the majority of the population. We've structured the delivery of contemporary medical care to center on the unusual procedures needed by only a minority of people. We've lost the close affiliation of physician and family that once saw the same doctor caring for perhaps two or three generations of a family. This means that the doctor to whom you're assigned by an HMO sees you as an office file, a quick glance through past notes that give minimal information about your health, and even less about your life. Should you still have a private practitioner, the chances are that she's been forced by economics to increase her patient load, so the time spent with you will concentrate on your recitation of symptoms, an exam, a prescription, perhaps a referral, and a hasty farewell, because the next patient is already in the adjoining examining room. Personal conversation, if any, covers the inanities of weather, work, or the like, with the patient offering few details about his overall health and life, and the physician not listening, anyway.

All this is in sharp contrast to the past, when there was little that the doctor could do for a patient other than being physically present at the bedside. Pharmaceuticals were limited. Surgery was often a last resort. What the doctor had to rely on was common sense and the personal knowledge of the patient, which could be acquired only from spending some important time with him. The practice of medicine was almost an art, not just a science.

In those days, the doctor would make house calls, seeing the patient in familiar surroundings. In this way, he'd gain a sense of the patient's family relationships, the cleanliness of the home, the types of food that were eaten, and whether or not there was stress from work. The doctor would learn about changes in the patient's life through questions about daily activities. "You used to like to walk into town for a beer each day, Harry," the doctor might say. "Your wife says you've stopped. She says you have her pick up a six-pack at the store, instead. I think you'd feel better if you'd start walking into town again every day. Maybe not for that beer—you're putting on a little gut—but you could stop by Mary's Café for some coffee."

It was like a conversation between two friends. Because the doctor knew his patient intimately, he could make valid suggestions for a modification in lifestyle. The doctor could also recognize whatever unhealthy habits other family members had that could affect the patient. Maybe the patient didn't smoke but someone else in the house did. The dangers of secondhand smoke (including free radicals, discussed in the following chapters) were not known, but it was sometimes suspected that smoking by any family member had a bad effect on all those who lived with that person. The doctor could talk to everyone in the house. "Your grandmother's having trouble catching her breath. Until she's doing better, it might be a good idea to air out her room and do your smoking outside. Take the cigarette out near the barn the way you did when you were a kid. It will take a few days to see any improvement, but I think we can keep her out of the county hospital and let her stay home, where she's happy. You could help her this way."

Today, the doctor may ascertain that the patient does not smoke but will rarely ask about a spouse, parent, sibling, or child in the same home. Since the patient is seen in the doctor's office, a nursing home, or a hospital, many problems are not evident. Worse, if smoking indoors is cited as a source of trouble, it is usually forbidden, in the form of an order: "There is to be no smoking in the house! You're killing your grandmother!" That, of course, makes the family members feel guilty or outraged, putting them on the defensive, as the gentle persuasion of the family physician never did.

Getting back to the case of "Harry," the same patient today would probably be given a medication for high blood pressure, another to lower cholesterol, and maybe a stimulant of some sort. The patient's exercising would continue to diminish. And the quality of the patient's life would decline, perhaps leading to an early death. All because the patient's past, his habits, and his home situation are unknown by the physician doing the treatment through contemporary delivery systems. And patients can no longer trust that they are their own best diagnosticians.

Women have fared worse than men. Not only are they

treated in the same manner as men, but for more than a century their health was the subject of myth and madness in medicine. (For example, in 1868 a leading gynecologist announced that if a girl of sixteen began dancing the polka, she would be sterile by the time she was twenty-one.) One of the factors contributing to their mistreatment was that women were expected to be sexually active whenever their men wanted them to be, and they were expected to turn out large numbers of children, because a big brood was seen as a guarantee of social security in rural America. Because many children died in their first five years, women kept having babies who, if they lived, would be able to care for the parents in old age.

What was not understood was that the number of children was not a problem. The fact is the "weaker sex" is far stronger than the male during the reproductive years. A premenopausal woman has greater stamina than a man, can endure more pain (by creating more easily the beta-endorphins needed to fight it). A woman who had ten children in her first fifteen years of marriage wasn't likely to be a health risk. Many such women carefully spaced the births and led long, productive lives. But when the man was too eager to return to intercourse immediately after childbirth and the woman was too compliant, there were health dangers. Trauma without recovery caused death or severe emotional problems. As it happened, many involved with the early efforts at birth control were women who had seen others have one baby every nine months and suffer the consequences. When Patrick Henry gave his famous "Give me liberty or give me death!" speech before the American Revolution, his insane wife was locked in the cellar while he was away from home. Few people knew it then, and few know it today. According to Peggy Eaton, wife of the Secretary of War during Andrew Jackson's administration and an early advocate of birth control, Mrs. Henry's madness was said to have been the result of pregnancy after pregnancy. Her body was given no chance to heal before she had intercourse and another baby.

Today, one of the accepted myths has to do with the odds against a woman's having heart disease. Women who have not yet reached menopause do, in fact, have biochemical protection, which is why an obese woman who smokes, eats high-cholesterol food, and has high blood pressure is not as likely as a man with similar risks to experience a heart attack until she's in her late forties or early fifties. He may have a heart attack five to ten years earlier. But the biochemical changes that occur during menopause level the playing field.

Tragically, although it is now well known, little is done about it. Women frequently have heart attacks, and often die before appropriate diagnoses are made. This is because women's symptoms are not so severe. If a woman's attack is not excruciatingly painful—and it rarely is—the appropriate countermeasures are not begun. Delayed diagnoses lead to a higher incidence of death and a lower utilization of appropriate care to reduce the severity and decrease the chance of a second, perhaps fatal heart attack.

Complicating the shoddy quality of much of the health care we receive today is our lack of attention to, and knowledge concerning, the way we treat and grow and process our food. The mistakes we continue to make in agriculture are as significant as those in health-care delivery.

For example, there was a time when I lived next to a large farm. One day, after a heavy rain, I walked toward the property line dividing my place from the farm. I noticed that the soil on my property was covered with earthworms. Normally, I didn't see many, since worms always dig through the soil, aerating it and helping crops grow naturally. The torrential rain, however, had flooded the ground, forcing the worms to the surface, where they began digging new holes.

When I glanced over at the farmer's property, I was surprised to see only mud. There were no earthworms, even though, just a few feet away, I had them everywhere. Curious, I mentioned this to my neighbor, and what he said was shocking.

"It's all the chemicals I use to treat the crops," the farmer told me, and began naming pesticides and other compounds meant to keep the crops from being reduced by insects and weeds. "The worms don't have a chance against them." And while most of us concerned with our health have reduced our consumption of red meat in favor of poultry and fish, we didn't do so because of our concern with chemicals added to the feed or other manmade problems. We did it because we understood the advantage of a diet more wholesome than the beef and potatoes that were the staple of many homes through the 1950s.

There are few problems with healthy birds raised naturally. Unfortunately, with the growing demand for poultry, the large national suppliers buy the millions of pounds of birds they need each week from small chicken ranchers. And it is the big suppliers who dictate how the birds will be raised. The subcontractors are now given growing times for the birds that are shorter than the time it takes a free-range (naturally raised) chicken to reach market weight. So, instead of wandering the grounds of the ranch, the birds stay in stacked holding pens, often never seeing daylight from the time of their birth until they are slaughtered. They are injected with antibiotics and growth hormones to make sure they do not become diseased in their unnatural quarters and that they will reach market weight more quickly. Since the buyers dominate the market, they stipulate the price per pound, and since it is more profitable to force-grow a bird in eight to ten weeks instead of the fourteen or more needed for free-range birds, the use of chemicals has become a given.

The result of this new type of chicken ranching is that the birds' bones are brittle, their joints frequently showing bruises and other damage. And the antibiotics and hormones remain in the meat after it is cooked, entering our bodies and adversely affecting our immune systems and metabolism.

What does this mean? First, there is a danger to all of us, especially our children, from the ingestion of growth hormones used in the chickens. We know that the switch of nursing infants from mother's milk to formula and cow's milk a generation or two ago was not good for the children's health. The mother's milk provides natural antibodies, appropriate growth hormones, and other essentials, enabling the nursing mother to give her newborn the healthiest possible start in life, a beginning that will benefit the child into adulthood. The cow's milk and formula given to bottle-fed children, however, have a biochemistry that is not normal for children and can create potential problems in the development of growth plates, bones, and muscles. The problems are subtle enough not to cause a backlash against the bottle, but what is right for the development of a calf that walks from birth is not necessarily right for the human child, who matures more slowly. Our ingestion of the growth hormones added to chickens just compounds the risks to our young.

The overdependency on antibiotics is even more dangerous. Every time you take medication to solve a health problem, the infection you're fighting tries all the harder to survive. It develops defenses against the antibiotics, so the more medication you use, the more likely it is that the antibiotic will soon be defeated by the mutating germs. And this is why antibiotics are no longer routinely prescribed for minor illnesses by knowledgeable physicians. But these very efforts to reduce antibiotic prescriptions are defeated when you ingest the antibiotics used in the raising of the chickens.

STEP 4: DON'T THROW OUT THE BABY WITH THE BATHWATER

Am I advocating that you abandon your doctor, do only self-diagnosis, and change your eating habits completely? Not at all. The ten natural remedies I advocate will certainly improve your health and possibly save your life, but they are not to be considered a substitute for a periodic checkup by your primary care physician, especially if you have problems that may be indicative of serious illness.

It is a matter of balance. Suppose, say, that you are a man with a prostate problem of some sort—a minor sexual dysfunction, frequent and occasionally painful urination—and you take saw palmetto, a natural remedy, that relieves the symptoms and eliminates the problem. You have no adverse side effects, no allergic reaction. And you have no need to boost your sex life artificially with an expensive and dangerous nostrum like Viagra.

Suppose, however, that the enlarged prostate problem, which can affect at least half of all men over fifty, is actually prostate cancer? The saw palmetto can still reduce or eliminate the symptoms, but there is only anecdotal evidence that it can aid in your full recovery. It may be necessary for you to have surgery or radiation treatment. Only if you have a regular periodic prostate exam will you know for certain the cause of your difficulty.

That is why you must understand your lifestyle. It is critical in assessing the symptoms that may prompt you to go to the doctor. This does not mean that you should fully trust your own diagnosis *or* that you should abdicate responsibility for treatment solely to the physician. Natural remedies are indeed the first line of defense for ensuring wellness. Natural remedies can prevent or cure most of the problems that physicians see in the course of the average day. But you must make certain that you are not that unusual individual with a problem that needs medical diagnosis. And you must remember that everyone needs a periodic medical evaluation in order to establish a baseline for health.

Remember, the best health comes when your physician is neither a god, to be revered above all else, nor a person to be dismissed because he or she lacks knowledge of natural remedies. Just be certain that you always listen first to the true expert on your body—yourself.

Now let's look at the ten natural remedies that can save your life, and learn why they've become necessities in our society.

Chapter Two

THE BASICS:
LIGHT, WATER, AND AIR

SOMETIMES WE MODERN HUMANS seem to do everything we can to ensure poor health. For thousands of years before our existence, people understood the rhythm of the planet. Holy books, like the Bible, tell us about the seasons of life, the time to plant, the time to nurture, the time to harvest. Our earliest ancestors, whether they were hunter-gatherers or stayed in one place to work the land, understood that survival called for three basic elements—light, water, and air. They worked when the sun shone. They slept when it was dark. They designed their living quarters so that they could avoid the pollution of cooking fires, and they sought clean water for drinking and bathing.

Of course they made mistakes. Anthropologists now know that there were cultures who overgrazed the land, creating seasons with little or no food; that there were times when poor farming methods or inappropriate sanitation contaminated what should have been clean drinking water. And some archeological remains show that the cave dweller did not always plan his living quarters in a way that kept him from inhaling smoke, which blackened both his lungs and his walls. But for the most part, these early people knew how to work with the three basics gifts of a healthy life.

Today we live in a world of denial, lauding a lifestyle because it is on the cutting edge of the electronic revolution. We've come to believe that anything involving computers and electronic communication must bring us into a new, better existence. The farm worker, although he may be essential to our survival, has as little to offer our understanding of health as the janitor in an office building has to offer the CEO of a major corporation. Some of the most highly paid employees in any business are those who are physically isolated, spending much of their day working at a keyboard and studying a monitor. We glorify the telecommuter, the person who each morning goes from bedroom to kitchen to whatever room holds the computer, modem, fax machine, and multiline telephone. We insist that our children become computer literate, going so far as to create summer camps where staying indoors to master computers is considered healthy recreation.

And what have we gained with the new lifestyle? We have one of the highest disposable per capita incomes in the world. Even the lowest-paid worker can realistically plan on owning a car so that he doesn't have to walk anywhere. Almost every adult in the nation owns a television set so that he can get his entertainment in the comfort of the living room, the bedroom, the kitchen, or the den. We buy video games so that we can play virtual basketball, run virtual races, and generally get a great workout on the video screen without worrying about "real time" sweat and heavy breathing. And then we look for the next big thing, the next adult toy we absolutely have to have because, despite our material possessions, we feel terrible much of the time.

Superficially, the effect of this great new existence has been a boost to the nation's economy. As I write, employment is at an all-time high, and many of the jobs are in retail sales. But there's a very visible dark side, one no one seems eager to discuss: that among the largest employers in any community are the hospitals, nursing homes, pharmacies, and other enterprises devoted to health care. The rust belt cities of Detroit, Cleveland, Akron, and Pittsburgh, where steel and automobile-related industries once dominated, now see health care as the major area of employment. The pay is often lower, but the number of jobs in health care far exceeds that in any other business.

And there's also been a sad and dramatic increase in drug use. I don't mean recreational drugs: illegal stimulants and depressants. I'm talking about pharmaceuticals that are so much a part of people's lives that they've become merely another course in a daily meal. Each night we consume an appropriate helping of meat, fish, or fowl, vegetables, fruit, whole grains, milk, Prozac, Valium, and, for dessert, our favorite sleeping pill. It's as though we've come to think of pills no longer as medicine, but as part of a healthy diet.

Once, people followed a hard day's work with a good night's rest. But no longer. Now we delight in our sleep deprivation, bragging about the hours we spend on the Internet or playing the latest video game.

We've reduced the overhead in our offices by sealing the windows for more efficient heating and cooling, and then cleverly used the floor space for cubicles without windows. Consequently, overhead has gone down and productivity has gone up. Except when our employees are out with colds. Or the flu. Or are slowed by mild depression, which limits their ability to function at full capacity.

Yes, we are technological wonders, able to turn day into night, night into day, and constantly in touch with the farthest corners of the room. Why is it, then, that we feel so terrible?

The answer is that we are in denial. We deny not only what we instinctively knew in years past, but we ignore current scientific knowledge regarding the quality of life we should demand for ourselves. That is why the first natural remedy I discuss is one of the most basic—light.

Active people have long considered night to be the enemy of their workaholic or playaholic existence. They may feel most fresh during the day, especially when they're out in the sun, but they also recognize that daytime brings responsibilities. They have to go to school or to their job. They have to do their shopping, care for their children. Daytime means the hustle and bustle of the daily routines. Night, for such people, is the time for adventure.

Let's look at bars and nightclubs. Dusk is called "happy hour," a transition from the artificial light of our offices, stores, and factories to the much dimmer artificial light of our favorite drinking and eating hangouts. Then, with darkness, come various forms of entertainment—disc jockeys, live bands, comedians, dancers—and the possibility of romance and seduction. With darkness comes the chance to play video games without keeping one eye out for the boss, or to enter chat rooms, where liars engage in sexual innuendo, the lonely create "friends" from words on a screen, and the obsessively curious explore topic after topic with their Web browsers.

Don't "night people" get tired? Of course they do. The pineal gland, a tiny manufacturing plant most people have never heard about, keeps pumping the natural sedative melatonin into the body. And with melatonin comes the promise of a good night's sleep, a sleep that combines rest with recovery from the stresses of daily life.

How does this denial of the need for rest affect our bodies? We age prematurely, experience depression, create immune deficiency and an increased susceptibility to illness, and construct other avoidable problems.

Even if we don't fight the natural rhythms of the body to the degree that friends and acquaintances may, our lifestyle poses risks we once could not have imagined happening to us, like cancer, heart disease, senescence, cataracts, and a host of other ailments. Well, maybe they were inevitable with old age. But not for us. Fortunately, we now know that a twofold natural remedy, one of the fundamental aspects of preventive medicine, can produce what people once would have labeled health miracles. Light and the hormone melatonin are perhaps the simplest yet most powerful natural remedies for saving our lives.

LIGHT

Your first concern is to gain adequate exposure to daylight or to its artificial near equivalent—full-spectrum light. In recent years, daylight has received the kind of bad press normally reserved for politicians, because exposure to the sun may cause premature aging and skin cancer, among other unwelcome conditions. And in the extreme, this is true. But just because water can drown a person in the middle of the ocean, we do not forget that it can save the life of someone wandering in the desert. Like water, the sun is essential to our well-being.

How essential? If you get too little of some wavelengths, your body will not properly absorb the nutrients from your food. Too little light, and you may suffer heart disease, stroke, fatigue, hair loss, cancer, hyperactivity, Alzheimer's disease, osteoporosis, or suppressed immune function.

The lack of sufficient full-spectrum light may be why some patients in hospitals and nursing homes have shorter lives and a poorer quality of life than people with similar conditions who stay home. Why? Because the homebound person is more likely to sit outside or go for a walk when he feels the need.

Even if the staff members of a hospital ward or nursing home are aware of the residents' need for regular daylight, the realities under which they work at the treatment facilities may make it impossible for them to provide it. Limited staffing means that patients cannot be moved about on a regular basis. Unless there's an open courtyard where the patients can be observed by staff members in case they need help, those patients' time in the sun will be limited, usually to two or three times a week. And because full-spectrum fluorescent bulbs of the type used in greenhouses are relatively expensive, the fixtures in institutions generally contain the traditional fluorescent bulbs or the equally bad incandescent bulbs.

We acknowledge that the sun does pose dangers. The ultraviolet spectrum of light is actually a form of radiation. But if you wear a hat, a long-sleeved shirt or blouse, use a high-number sunblock (#45 is usually the highest number available and is well worth the cost), wear sunglasses that offer little tinting but good UVA and UVB protection, and limit your time outside, you will receive most of the sun's benefits and incur few adverse effects. Exposure to daylight is so important that you must try to get out every day, even if it means taking time during a lunch break when you don't happen to have all the protective clothing or sunscreen. In these instances, just remember to practice moderation.

The negative effects of too little light have become part of a folk culture in this age of the computer. We've all heard tales of obsessive computer lovers, people who work high-tech jobs and spend hours mastering computer languages. They sit alone in darkened rooms, with only the monitor for light, designing software, eliminating "bugs" from new products, and communicating with friends and other "geeks" throughout the world. They rarely socialize with flesh-and-blood people. They tend to overeat, often surviving on caffeine-based soft drinks and junk food, getting truly nutritious meals on an irregular basis. They're tired, and soon find themselves most comfortable when entering data or typing messages. E-mail is not just a tool for communication for these people; they've become so psychologically isolated that it doesn't occur to them to pick up a telephone.

It is edifying to compare the lifestyle of the mythic computer user with that of the person afflicted with seasonal affect disorder (SAD). SAD sufferers have the seasonal problem of depression. The fewer the number of daylight hours, the more difficulty they have in getting through the day. This is why SAD is most common in northern cities, where the winter's daylight hours are brief and often overcast, and the weather often so blustery that many people choose to stay indoors. But at least SAD sufferers get relief when the days are long and they get out in the sun; their experience during long days of darkness is the year-round experience of the computer geeks in self-imposed isolation.

What are the common symptoms of seasonal affect disorder? A tendency to withdraw from others, to overeat, and to grow tired—the same traits that are typical of the personality of the computer addict. Yet as long as the computer user meets corporate deadlines or otherwise contributes to her job, we don't think about her unhealthy lifestyle or problems. I suspect, though, that in a few years we'll see a disproportionate number of immune system disorders in the diehard computer user. In large part because she's not getting adequate sunlight.

YOU AND THE LIGHT
AND THE MELATONIN

Our bodies, and presumably the bodies of all living creatures, work most efficiently when attuned to the lightness-darkness cycle. Exposure to bright light is like a wall switch that regulates body chemistry. Turn on the bright light, and we go about our jobs rapidly and effectively. Athletes reach peak performance. Office workers think clearly and effectively. Scientists refine their discoveries. Students learn more easily. And people performing potentially dangerous activities, like driving cars, operating heavy equipment, flying airplanes, or loading and unloading trucks, have far fewer accidents than do their co-workers on later shifts.

Darkness turns the switch off, and we lose our alertness. Our judgment falters, our reactions are slower, we think less clearly, and we may feel a touch of sadness or melancholy, even though we've enjoyed a happy and productive day. Those who try to extend their waking hours by going to bars and nightclubs often find themselves meditative and quiet or boisterous and uninhibited. The former is related to the need for sleep; the latter to the dwindling of common sense caused by an inability to think clearly. And neither is good.

These emotional changes are biochemical shifts controlled by the pineal gland. This gland, which slows down and eventually stops working as we age, produces one of the vital chemicals in your body—melatonin. When you understand how to work properly with light, and when to supplement your natural melatonin, you may discover that you feel better than you have in years. You'll also find that the ravages of aging, like cataracts, are slowed, eliminated, or, in some instances, partly healed.

The basic requirement for the functioning of a healthy pineal gland, during those years when it is at peak performance, is lots of light during the day and the avoidance of bright lights at night. Sound simple? It is. Do we follow the rule? Rarely.

Windows, strongly tinted eyewear, automobile windshields, and all the devices that let light into our offices, homes, and lives reduce the quality of that light. By the time the light passes through an office window, it usually lacks the desirable full spectrum. People who have long commuting times may think they're getting sun, but the value of the sunlight is dangerously diminished. Much good does come from added brightness, but brightness is not the only quality of the light you need to receive during each twenty-four-hour cycle. It is critical that you expose yourself directly to the sun each day; if you have to be inside, make sure that your body receives full-spectrum bright light.

The ideal office would be run like an elementary school on a warm spring day, when both students and teachers are restless. First, the classroom door is open; there are no isolating cubicles. Next, the windows are large, letting in bright light and, sometimes, fresh air, eliminating the glass "filter" the light has to pass through. And third, the children have a recess two and sometimes three times a day. They're sent out to play in the morning. They're sent out to play in the afternoon. And occasionally they're sent outside during lunchtime. The result is a group of happy, productive children who are at the peak of their abilities during the day and sleep well at night.

But the modern office environment is not like that, and it must be countered by a distinct change in lifestyle. This is easiest to bring about if you're one of the growing number of telecommuters, working from home. Still, you can make effective changes if you work in an office.

1. If you drive to work, do not park your car in the parking garage for your building or in a nearby lot. Park it at least a half mile away and walk to work. This may add from five to ten minutes to your commuting time, but you'll almost always spend those minutes in the daylight.

   If you take public transportation, get off two or three stops before or after your usual stop and then walk the rest of the way. Again, you'll gain a few minutes of daylight exposure.

2. Take a daily break and go outside. This may be during your lunch hour or during coffee breaks. Oddly, office workers who smoke are doing their bodies a limited favor when, following the rules, they go outside to light up. As it turns out, the health codes meant to protect nonsmoking workers from secondhand smoke actually help the smokers themselves by sending them outside. But remember that going outside and *not* smoking is far better!

3. Equip your home with bright lights on dimmer switches. The brighter the light, the more healthy it is. The dimmer switch lets you adjust the light to meet the growing darkness of night. You'll be able to see, read, and do everything you normally do, but you'll be using the decreasing light to mimic nature and allow the pineal gland to begin its

nightly production of melatonin. Having full-spectrum light is also best whenever and wherever possible.

4. Working a third shift is unavoidable for many health-care workers, law enforcement officers, and manufacturing plant employees, but these people must restructure their lives to create a natural environment. Take advantage of the bright light your job allows you, if possible. If it doesn't allow bright light, then plan your sleep schedule around periods when you can have extensive exposure to it.

On the other hand, you can turn your bedroom into an artificial night chamber. Place blackout curtains on the windows. If you can't find them in a store, get opaque black fabric that will block the light. Stores that stock supplies for professional photographers may provide you with such material, since it's used in darkrooms that have windows.

If you can't sew the curtains, have someone else make them. Or just cover your bedroom windows with the fabric and seal the corners with gaffer's tape, a kind of duct tape used by photographers and available at many camera stores. You can then cover the fabric with attractive curtains, the most opaque ones you find. Using a sleeping mask is also a good idea, since keeping your eyes from seeing the light will help alter your biological clock to match your odd working shift.

5. Bright light is critical regardless of its spectrum. Take advantage of windows. The closer you can work to a source of bright light, the better. If you have a choice between a cubicle arrangement and offices where the employees can sit near windows, the windows should win every time.

Some employers fear that their employees will daydream, staring out the glass. While this may occur, the slight decrease in productivity is offset by the major increase in the benefits of exposure to light. Unfortunately, too often in corporate America efficient use of space takes precedence over the health of the workers.

THE PINEAL GLAND

Earlier, I mentioned melatonin, the hormone that is necessary to the body's proper use of light. Melatonin is created in the digestive tract, but as we saw, the pineal gland acts as its chemical switch.

The eyes are crucial to the functioning of the pineal gland. When we wake in the morning and light hits our eyes, some of us leap out of bed, fully awake, with a song in our hearts. But some of us drag ourselves out of bed, cursing the brightness and wondering how anyone could be civil before noon. Either way, once light has hit our eyes, the pineal gland shuts down the production of melatonin, so even the groggiest of morning risers are biochemically pushed into full wakefulness.

The process reverses itself when darkness falls. As your eyes sense the lack of light, your pineal gland begins manufacturing fresh melatonin. You become relaxed and sleepy while your body prepares for rest and recovery from the day. This recovery reaches a peak at the darkest hour of the morning, around two or three A.M.

The effects of the melatonin are hampered, to a degree, by activity. Someone who likes to go partying, to close bars and nightclubs, is challenging his melatonin to overcome his desire to stay awake. And third-shift workers, who are rarely in bright light, also work against their bodies' biochemistry. That's why most one-car accidents *not* involving alcohol, drugs, or any-thing else that would impair judgment occur between 3 A.M. and 4:30 A.M. At that point the driver's melatonin level is at the point where sleep is an overwhelming requirement of the body and the exhausted driver crashes.

Recently, melatonin has become known throughout the country as nature's sleeping pill. Publications run stories about melatonin's value in resetting our biological clocks, and trav-elers are exhorted to use melatonin when crossing time zones, because a melatonin supplement taken approximately an hour before you go to sleep will reset your body in much the same way that you reset your watch. Although the use of melatonin as a natural sleeping pill and corrector of your biological clock does make it important to your health, its primary role as a life-saving remedy lies in its other attributes.

Melatonin, especially in its role as an antioxidant, appar-ently slows or prevents some of the common illnesses attendant on aging. The trouble is, the older we get, the less melatonin is manufactured by our pineal gland, and the faster we can deteri-orate. The pineal gland routinely begins to fail when we turn forty to fifty years old, and it continues to wane until there is no measurable output of melatonin. Supplementation reverses this process. This means that when an adult begins taking melatonin supplements, his quality of life will be improved and the dan-gers of serious illness will be decreased. Lack of melatonin con-tributes dramatically to the onset of senescence, the degenera-tion of Alzheimer's, the spread of numerous cancers, and other problems.

You will see the term "antioxidant" frequently throughout this book. Its role is to neutralize the negative effects of free radicals, another term you will often see here.

FREE RADICALS

The term "free radical" sounds like something you once read about in the news accounts of demonstrations in China, when supporters of jailed dissidents demanded their freedom. In fact, the biological "free radical" is something that can be corrosive and damaging to your health. The term itself is relatively new. Until 1969, biologists believed that diseases came from outside our bodies. They attacked us through our pores, mouths, and nasal passages. They were not manufactured within us, as had been suggested by Dr. Denham Harman, a pioneering researcher in the field. He was scoffed at for thinking that both diseases and aging could be caused by internal processes, as well as by external assaults on the body. Fifteen years after he postulated his "heresy" concerning free radicals, however, we began to understand what he meant. And today we not only know the truth, but we have ways to deal with the problem.

The discovery, in 1969, was so technical that it gained little or no attention in the popular press. Scientists working with red blood cells isolated a copper protein that had no known function, and on further study, they ascertained that it was an enzyme uniting two superoxide radicals. These free radical components are necessary for the normal utilization of oxygen (which is what led to their discovery). Free radicals can activate hormones and start reactions that destroy bacteria and viruses. And if we could keep them at such tasks, they would cause no problems.

But they have their bad side. They can, for instance, inhibit the white blood cells' production of disease-fighting organisms. They've been compared to rust on a car. Exposed to rock salt and similar destructive materials, the car will, over time, be destroyed. Once the metal is exposed, rust spots appear and grow and eventually make holes in the metal, ultimately separating the body from the frame.

Bad free radicals attack the covering of the cell membrane, which shields your essential DNA from outside assault. And once the DNA is in jeopardy, the damaged cells are unable to divide and reproduce. The body, then, is at greater risk of arthritis, heart disease, cancer, and other disorders we once assumed were a "natural" part of aging. If you're young when the free radicals assault your DNA, you may even pass the damage on to the next generation during your pregnancy.

Unfortunately, we have to expose ourselves to dangerous free radicals in order to obtain the good free radicals. For example, ultraviolet rays from the sun naturally cause the creation of bad free radicals. Yet if we don't get sufficient sunlight each day, our immune system is endangered. The pineal gland may not produce enough melatonin to help our bodies ward off disease and delay the degenerative aspects of aging.

We can control our exposure to natural free radicals by such simple precautions as wearing sunblock and eyeglasses with lenses that keep out UV (ultraviolet light). But the unnatural causes of free radicals demand that we change our lifestyle. Among the unnatural causes of bad free radicals are inhaled and secondhand cigarette smoke, and though many scientists debate whether secondhand smoke is actually responsible for pulmonary and cardiovascular diseases, there is no doubt that it creates negative free radicals. The question is not *if* each of us will be affected, but *how*.

Other sources of free radical damage are alcohol, pesticides, radiation, herbicides, solvents, asbestos, wood smoke, ozone, and sulfur dioxide. In other words, even if you live an idyllic suburban existence, with a large yard, plenty of trees, and a garden where you grow some of your vegetables, you may be in trouble. The pesticides you use to protect your crops, the grill on which you prepare food in the summer, the materials you rely on to maintain your home, and the drinks you enjoy on your patio while watching the sun set can all expose you to free radical damage.

How serious is this? A few years ago the *New York Times* reported that in Russia, an industrialized nation with few environmental controls, the life expectancy for the average man was 57.3 years, fourteen years fewer than for a man in the United States. And one reason is thought to be his high exposure to dangerous free radicals caused by indifference to pollutants and other irritants. This is also why environmentalists question the irradiation of food and the substitution of chemicals for fat and other elements in our diet. They fear, in part, a rise in dangerous forms of free radicals.

ANTIOXIDANTS

This destabilization of healthy molecules is called oxidative stress and is the most frequent cause of brain damage. In fact, at this writing many researchers believe that oxidative stress may be the primary cause of Alzheimer's. Even if that does not prove to be accurate, it is true that oxidative stress does exacerbate and hasten conditions like Alzheimer's.

Brain damage is readily noticed because the brain is the largest organ to require oxygen molecules for proper functioning. If you, however, have experienced one of the various forms of cancer, cataracts, heart disease, or a host of other seemingly unrelated problems, the chances are that you're a victim of free radicals. Even one of the so-called ravages of aging, like wrinkled skin, is in large measure caused by free radicals. Note how often people who smoke cigarettes, cigars, and pipes develop more youthful-looking skin after they've stopped smoking for a few months.

Obviously, it's critical to reduce the forms of free radicals caused by humans. But no matter how serious our efforts to do so, it will take many years to achieve measurable results. In the meantime, we have to rely on antioxidants, the molecules that serve as electron donors. Their function is to stabilize the body's free radical molecules without hurting the healthy molecules. And how do you get antioxidants into your body? Just as your mother said: Eat your fruits and vegetables.

All right. So it isn't quite that simple in contemporary America, where our food doesn't go from our garden to the dinner table. Fresh fruits and vegetables must be eaten as part of a healthful diet, but they can be supplemented by those nutrients that are the primary sources of antioxidants: the hormone melatonin and the common vitamin supplements—A, C, and E. In this section, we'll concentrate on melatonin and its antioxidant properties.

Oxygen, like water, is both good and bad. A real paradox! Oxygen is burned by the body to create energy and a variety of by-products in a manner not unlike wood burned for heat. Light a log and you will be able to keep warm through a cold night, cook your food, and keep away many dangerous animals if you are camping. You will also have smoke rising from the flames, and the smoke will irritate your eyes, nose, throat, and lungs while damaging the atmosphere.

The by-products of the body's burning of oxygen are called reactive oxygen species, or ROS. This is the equivalent of the bad portion of wood smoke.

ROS are what we have been calling free radicals. There is an unpaired electron in the free radical's outer orbit causing it to want to steal another electron or even another hydrogen atom.

The end result will be one of several possibilities. The ROS might break through the protective cell wall, or the ROS might take a tiny bit of DNA from the cell's nucleus, or it might cause damage to the cell's energy source, altering the chemistry of what is known as the mitrochondria.

A single ROS is damaging. What makes this problem of concern to us is that millions of free radicals are created every second within the body.

The antioxidants neutralize bad free radicals by changing their molecular structure. If you have a sufficient supply of anti-oxidants in your body, free radical damage will be minimized, and your health will be improved.

We'll see later in the book how many of the natural reme-dies that will save your life are antioxidants or agents that stim-ulate the antioxidant defense against free radicals. Research has shown that medicine in the twenty-first century will rely more and more on the properties of antioxidants, and less and less on pharmaceuticals. This, of course, is one reason the pharmaceu-tical companies have been engaging in intensive media cam-paigns to sell directly to the consumer. You've seen the ads: Speak to your doctor about this drug or that one for some common ailment. What you've not been told is that, though these drugs may work well, they can also encourage the bad free radicals in your body. Unless a pharmaceutical treatment is absolutely critical, you will fare better with natural remedy al-ternatives to make the necessary body chemistry changes with-out adding bad free radicals to your system.

It's a little like the heartworm medications sold for dogs. The medication is a poison that, in higher dosages, would kill the dog, but the manufacturer keeps the dose so low that the heartworms are killed first. The medication is stopped after the death of the worms and before the dog is endangered, but not before the dog has had a low-level poison added to its body.

In some instances, given our present state of knowledge, there may be few alternatives to pharmaceuticals. The more we learn about natural remedies that have proved safe and effective for centuries, the sooner we'll be able to cut back on the use of these pharmaceuticals. And perhaps one day our present "state of the art" dependency on pharmaceuticals, and the unwillingness of many physicians to consider natural remedies, will be considered incompetent health care.

LIGHT AND MELATONIN

Now that you better understand antioxidants, free radicals, your pineal gland and the melatonin it produces, and your body's utilization of light, let's look at the first natural remedy.

LIGHT

Daylight and its near equal, full-spectrum light, are essential to disease prevention and healing. No matter what's wrong with you or what may go wrong in the future, you will call on light as an element in your healing.

Use light every day in the ways that best serve your pineal gland. Have full-spectrum lightbulbs in as many rooms as possible. (These can be fluorescent tubes or bulbs to be used like traditional incandescents.) Have dimmer switches on the lights, where they are appropriate, so that you can keep them bright during the day and subdued at night.

Open your curtains and shades, letting the sun shine in as

much as possible. Get outside to walk in the daylight, even in bad weather.

Your eyes will need UVA and UVB (the two different forms of light) protection, but that doesn't mean heavily tinted sunglasses. You want the full spectrum of the light, eliminating only the potentially damaging ultraviolet rays.

Use daylight as a stimulant. If you're in an office, factory, school, or other indoor setting most of the time, take breaks and go outside. Even five minutes of walking in the daylight will serve as an emotional stimulant.

Take at least a twenty-minute brisk walk in daylight every day. If that's not possible, try alternative exercise possibilities (an exercise bicycle or treadmill) at home in a room with full-spectrum, bright light for the room.

The exercise will strengthen your cardiovascular system, enhance your lungs, and improve your ability to fight bad free radicals. And it will act as a natural tranquilizer, leaving you both invigorated and calm.

MELATONIN SUPPLEMENTS

An hour or two before bedtime is when you should take melatonin supplements. The light in your home is now dimmer than it was during the day. If you're young enough to have a fully functioning pineal gland, the dim light will enhance the natural production of the hormone. If your pineal gland is failing or has stopped functioning, the supplements will help recreate the youthful actions that will prolong your health. This means that your biological clock will be functioning, ensuring you a proper night's sleep even if you've shifted time zones during a cross-country or international trip. You'll be keeping your cholesterol and blood pressure at normal levels, reducing your risk of heart disease. And most important, you'll be restoring your immune system.

Much of the body's healing work is done while you sleep, which is why people who are sick need extra rest. Preliminary research indicates that sleep, coupled with melatonin supplements, is likely to help your body's immune system destroy cells that might otherwise lead to cancer, especially of the breast and the prostate.

Melatonin also acts as a cleansing and sharpening agent for the brain. Nerve cells, which deteriorate as we age in part because of the decline in the pineal gland hormone production, are strengthened by the melatonin. It also aids in the creation of alternative pathways for nerve cells so that the old pathways are not overloaded.

And if you're regularly exposed to electromagnetic field radiation (EMF), you'll get another benefit from melatonin. There are several sources of EMF to one degree or another, among them computer monitors and television sets, as well as high-voltage power lines. In fact, for years the power industry has been under the scrutiny of ranchers and farmers, who often share large open lands with power grids and high-voltage lines. There is some evidence that EMF affects the health of the cattle grazing in these areas and the people living there. So far, however, the evidence has been anecdotal, and conclusive studies have not yet been completed.

It may come as a surprise that EMF is a problem with electric blankets. (These are popular with couples whose sleeping habits are different, because many blankets have two heat settings, one for each spouse). The trouble is that the blankets wrap the sleepers in an EMF field for eight hours a day.

Although no one yet knows the specific dangers posed by

EMF, there is growing concern that it may reduce the body's production of melatonin. This would account for the less effective immune system in people exposed to the field. I believe that the EMF problem can be countered through melatonin supplements.

Perhaps most important is the relation between melatonin and aging. All of us look for the Fountain of Youth that Ponce de León once sought in the region now known as Florida. He was hoping to find a spring of life-giving water that would erase the ravages of aging. Personally, I think the difference between a person of one hundred and one of twenty-five should be measured by the wisdom of the accumulated years, not by the body's deterioration. All of us, however, want to make the years we have as healthy and productive as possible, which is why we should pay attention to melatonin. It strengthens the immune system, reduces or eliminates the dangers from cataracts, keeps our minds sharp, and generally allows for a richer, fuller life. Without melatonin, your quality of life would be lower, and there is the chance of premature death from illnesses that are preventable.

SIDE BENEFITS

Melatonin stimulates the body's production of three key hormones—testosterone, estrogen, and adrenaline—all of them critical factors in your sex life. Thus, one pleasant side effect of melatonin supplementation is the maintenance of a healthy sex drive or the restoration of a declining sex drive.

Can this save your life? I know of adolescent boys who try to convince adolescent girls that somehow sex is essential for good health. And in the late 1770s and 1780s, when Benjamin Franklin was working for the Colonists in Passy, France, he used similar reasoning for his seductions. The brilliant states-man, inventor, and publisher, who was also an outrageous womanizer into his seventies, wrote to a woman in Passy that when he was young and the ladies all agreed to go to bed with him, he was in perfect health. Now, he explained, he was bothered by gout, because the object of his affection refused to have sex with him. It was therefore important that this woman go to bed with him to improve his health.

The attempt wasn't successful, but there was some validity to the request. One factor in health is a committed relationship. Studies have shown that loving couples have a longer life and fewer health problems than those who live alone. The physical side of marriage, coupled with the emotional commitment, gives a boost to your immune system. Thus, what may sound solely hedonistic is as important for your health as it is enjoyable.

PRECAUTIONS

Many medications are concocted to mimic the body's natural chemistry. There are pharmaceuticals aimed at strengthening the immune system, increasing the production of hormones, lowering blood pressure, and doing all the other things that melatonin does in a natural manner. If you take both, melatonin and medications, there is a chance that your body will be receiving what amounts to an overdose. This is also true of such mood-altering medications as Prozac and Valium. Even the regular use of aspirin can be a problem.

If you're taking melatonin and no other medications, and your doctor suggests you take a pharmaceutical, tell him about the melatonin. In some instances, the melatonin, perhaps in an elevated dose, will be sufficient. I recommend 1 to 2 milligrams as a basic dose for people age forty to sixty. Some elderly individuals need more, but never more than 5 milligrams. In other instances, you and your doctor may feel that the pharmaceutical is of short-term importance, in which case you should briefly stop the melatonin, or use less each day, or have your doctor regularly examine you for problems. Always check with your doctor, and cross-check with your pharmacist. Many pharmacists are more knowledgeable than physicians in such matters.

Additionally, use great caution and work closely with your doctor before taking melatonin supplements if you're nursing a baby, have fertility problems, or suffer from hormonal disorders, depression or another psychiatric disorder, cancer, autoimmune disorders, or allergies. While melatonin may help prevent some unwanted diseases and conditions, it may interfere with some treatments.

Children and adolescents (through the age of twenty-five) should *never* take melatonin.

It is doubtful that anyone needs regular supplements before he reaches the age of forty. The one exception is the traveler (the international pilot or flight attendant) who regularly crosses time zones. If this pertains to you, discuss melatonin as a sleep aid and biological clock adjuster with your physician. And never hesitate to use a sleep aid like a mask to block out light from your eyes. You may think you look like a character in an old Western, but if it helps the pineal gland's on-off switch to work well, it's worth it.

WATER

As we saw earlier, the first three basic alternative therapies are the basics: light, water, and air. Light is by far the most complex. What we've learned in recent years has come as a surprise to researchers and a boon to all of us concerned with our health.

Water is less complex. We need water to survive. Our bodies are 70 percent water. At any given time, adults have approximately sixteen gallons of water in their systems. If we don't replenish our supply within two or three days, we will almost certainly die. We can go without food for a month or longer. We can go without light, though we'll pay some health penalties for an indefinite time. But going without water for just a few days means death.

There was a time when we physicians would simply tell our patients to drink a lot of water—say eight eight-ounce glasses a day—and believe we had given good advice. Today we know better. Not only does everyone's need for water increase with age, for reasons we don't yet fully understand, but our nation's water supply has become increasingly toxic. Almost all water has to be specially treated before it can be safely consumed, and the treatment itself may pose subtle risks. All of us should know this!

THE DANGERS

It was in 1988 that the U.S. Department of Public Health first undertook the study of water contamination and found that 85 percent of water in the United States is contaminated to some degree. The cause may be human and animal waste, or chlorine, fluoride, and toxic ammonia, additives meant to purify the water or improve its quality. In addition, because of the heedless way in which we treat our water supply, some cities, including the largest in the nation, have water with as many as five hundred different parasites, viruses, and bacteria, each one capable of making you sick.

One of these, the pathogen cryptosporidium, has been mentioned in newspaper stories of contaminated water in major cities over the years. Milwaukee, Wisconsin, made headlines in 1993 when the illnesses of 370,000 residents and the deaths of 142 were believed to be directly connected to the contamination. Six confirmed outbreaks between 1986 and 1996 caused more than seven million people to suffer diarrhea, dehydration, severe stomach cramping, and the risk of death—all this because of a single-cell parasite that could easily have been removed from the water with a good home purification system. (WARNING! There are many water-purification systems on the market, each making claims of great value. Most, however, are of limited value, and even some of the better ones do not provide all the protection you may need. I once took a look at a number of models of the 4.6 million home purification systems sold in the United States in 1994—the manufacturers' information broke them down by type, which made the task much simpler than it sounds—and found that fewer than one in ten could prevent cryptosporidium from entering your body.)

Another contaminant frequently found in water, according to studies done at the Massachusetts Institute of Technology, is *Helicobacter pylori,* believed to contribute to stomach ulcers and stomach cancers.

Even cities using well water and other forms of groundwater have faced difficulties. In some cases, once desirable manufacturing plants create more problems than benefits. You may have read that the computer-chip industry has been leaving California's so-called Silicon Valley for other regions. There are some sound business reasons for the move, but one certain factor is that the manufacture of computer chips and similar equipment is both water-intensive and water-polluting. The waste from the work has been dumped, for years, in a manner that allowed it to leach into rivers, streams, and other waterways. In several instances, the contamination became so serious that it was cheaper for the firm to relocate than to clean up the mess. But those who stay behind face long-term illness!

In Tucson, Arizona, almost two decades ago, a manufacturing plant was contaminating the well water. Veterinarians were the first to notice the problem, because they were treating dogs with kidney stones and other disorders they knew were related to the drinking water. Because the physiology of the pets was similar to that of humans, the observation served as a warning to the citizens of Tucson to use distilled water for drinking and cooking.

In recent years it has been found that hospitals, pharmaceutical companies, and other businesses using substances that leave low-level radioactive waste have been dumping that waste into the sewers. This is not a secret plot. The companies were acting in accordance with antiquated laws that allowed a certain level of such dumping. Now that we know the waste has been entering public water supplies, however, we also know that the cumulative volume can be dangerous to health. Yet parts of our country continue to be plagued by these problems.

It is doubtful that you can find any water supply entirely free of pollutants that contribute to cancer and other degenerative diseases. These contaminated waters are a major source of free radicals in the body. And their dangers are compounded by the plumbing itself.

Years ago, doctors noted a high incidence of lead poisoning in homes where there were no lead-based paints and no utensils or serving dishes decorated with lead-based paint were being used. What they discovered was that the lead poisoning could be traced to the lead in the composition of pipes and in the joint solder in the pipes. Thankfully, this problem has generally been remedied.

Less deadly but more insidious is the problem of depression noticed in such cities as New York, where copper plumbing has been used for years. The trouble is that old copper pipes gradually erode, allowing traces of copper to leach into the water and be consumed in amounts far more than we need.

This extra copper caused mild depression. People found themselves lacking enthusiasm in their personal and professional lives and feeling lethargic. They were sad when they had no reason to be. The experience was bewildering, and it was not eased by doctors who prescribed mood-altering pharmaceuticals. It was only when the drinking water was changed, eliminating the trace amounts of copper in excess of the body's needs, that people felt better.

In fact, if you live in one of the older cities in the East or Midwest, there is the chance that some of the water you consume contains an excess of copper from aging pipes. It may not be enough copper to discolor the water or alter its taste, and it may not be enough to cause illness. But it may well be enough to leave you with a mild depression, and depression, we have seen, contributes to immune-system deficiency.

Despite these hazards, drinking large quantities of water each day is essential. And I mean water, not just liquids. Many people substitute fruit juice, coffee, tea, and other beverages for water, not realizing that even if the drink is healthful and nutritious, it is not a substitute for water. Maybe it will quench your thirst for a while, but it won't lubricate your body's moving parts or fulfill water's job of handling the processes of digestion, absorption, and elimination. It won't transport nutrients throughout your body, dilute toxins, and remove wastes and poisons, as pure water will.

Most people suffer mild dehydration during the day without ever realizing it, because they quench their thirst with other liquids. Yet if you suffer from colds, fatigue, constipation, arthritis, kidney disease, circulatory diseases, and even frontal headaches, you may be lacking adequate water. Although that lack may not be the only factor, it is so important that the simple reality is that the more water you drink each day—and consider the eight eight-ounce glasses to be the absolute minimum as you age—the healthier you will be.

TYPES OF WATER

Hard Water: Hard water has a high concentration of the minerals calcium and magnesium. It has a distinctive taste and it prevents soap from lathering easily. You'll find a filmy sediment on everything you wash, from your clothing to your hair.

Some studies show that regions with hard water have a reduced incidence of heart disease, but these studies are inconclusive and run counter to the potential negative effect of calcium on the heart, arteries, and bones. (NOTE: Calcium ingested through your food has a positive effect on the bones and vascular system. It deposits the calcium inside the bones, helping to build and strengthen them. Calcium and other minerals coming from hard water deposits are left outside the bones. This is not beneficial.)

Soft Water: Soft water comes in two forms. The first is naturally soft. The second is hard water that has been treated for the removal of the calcium and magnesium. Unfortunately, that treatment also results in the deterioration of pipes. Depending upon the type of plumbing, the treatment to artificially soften water can cause copper, zinc, iron, arsenic, lead, and cadmium to get into the water. The greatest danger comes from the galvanized pipes found in some older buildings. But no form of artificially softened water is as safe as the hard water or naturally soft water found in most communities.

Tap Water: Many of us have the expectation that tap water is clean and safe. The treatment of our water systems is a primary use of our tax dollars. And many water workers take great pride in the quality of the drinking water they produce through the various cleansing steps to which they subject the water before it comes out of our faucets. There are, however, many factors outside their control. In fact, in just two years, 1994 and 1995, the Natural Resources Defense Council found that 45 million Americans, utilizing 18,500 different water systems, were drinking water so contaminated that 900,000 people were sickened and 100 died.

Part of the problem is that clean water standards for communities are usually based on individual quantities of each type of contaminant: You may have so many parts of contaminant A and so many of contaminant B. What is not factored in is what the *total* accumulation of these dangerous substances can do to put you at a high health risk.

Take chlorine as an example. The addition of chlorine to drinking water at the turn of the century greatly improved its safety compared with the water available before its use. We now know, however, that the quantities of chlorine used vary not only by community but sometimes within the same community. And while it does kill disease-causing bacteria, its by-products, we've recently learned, can cause cancer. Since the risk varies with the amount of chlorine, the Environmental Protection Agency is now considering setting a maximum quantity of chlorine that can be used in order to better protect the population. It is uncertain, though, whether the reduced risk of cancer that should result will be offset by increased risk of bacterial contamination.

Fluoridation: Perhaps you're old enough to remember the controversy in the 1950s revolving around the addition of fluoride to drinking water. Fluoride is and has long been known to be a poison, but it is also a chemical that protects teeth from decay. That is why it is added to many brands of toothpaste and why dentists suggest fluoride treatments for children and often for adults. In fact, fluoride is found naturally in some water sources, one of the facts that original proponents of fluoridation for all water supplies used to justify the addition.

Today, after many years of our drinking fluoridated water, no long-term studies have linked fluoridated water with stronger bones and teeth. Instead, there have been indications of links to damaged and mottled teeth, as well as to health problems like osteomalacia and osteoporosis.

Additionally, recent attention has been focused on the way that fluoride is added to water supplies. Often, the fluoridation method is the addition of two salts, sodium fluoride and fluorosalicylic acid, which are industrial by-products, not elements found in nature. When they're not being used to "help" our water supply, they are incorporated into such commercial products as insecticides and rat poisons. The quantities are markedly different, of course, but it's obvious that the real value is in the damage these salts can cause, not the benefits. In fact, there is some evidence of a higher than normal incidence of Down syndrome and cancer in some communities with a higher than average amount of fluoridation.

Consequently, I believe we should cease to fluoridate water. Each of us has a unique physiology, and even if we determined the safe addition of fluoride for any one person, finding a standard for the thousands or millions who live in our cities is impossible. Safety is relative to the individual.

Mineral Water: Mineral water is natural spring water quite popular in Canada and Europe. When it is bottled, the bottling must be done at the source of free-flowing water (neither pumped nor forced up from the ground). It contains minerals, although the amounts vary with the source. Thus it is good if you experience a mineral deficiency, but only if you choose water from a spring that contains the mineral or minerals you need. Since the minerals are not listed on the label, you can learn this only through costly analysis. Even worse, some mineral water provides an excess of minerals you do not need, and drinking it can have harmful side effects such as edema, hypertension, and congestive heart failure from too much sodium.

Mineral waters are usually carbonated. This has led to bottlers of soda waters and sparkling waters to call some of their drinks mineral waters once they add sodium phosphates, bicarbonates, and citrates. Since these merchants actually start with tap water that has gone through a distilling process or water that has been specially filtered, their products are not the same as natural mineral water.

Natural Spring Water: This is familiar to most of us who walk past a bottled water cooler. When the suppliers say that the product is "natural," all they mean is that the mineral content has not been altered. What they don't tell you is whether the water has been filtered or otherwise treated. They also don't tell you the source—and often the word "spring" does not mean that it came from a free-flowing spring.

To be legal, spring water is any water that rises naturally to the earth's surface from an underground reservoir. Usually it is good, but some reservoirs are contaminated. Then, too, many contaminate the water by not properly cleaning the cooler through which it runs. A proper cleaning requires that at least once a month a mixture of equal quantities of hydrogen peroxide and baking soda is run through the reservoir and spigots. Following that, at least four or five gallons of tap water should be run through to rinse the system clean. Only then should a new bottle be placed on the cooler. Otherwise, bacteria will build up, adding another risk.

A variation of natural spring water is sparkling water, usually sold either as natural sparkling water or as carbonated natural water. The natural sparkling water is carbonated at its source; its mineral content has not been altered. Carbonated natural water has been carbonated away from the source.

Unnatural Water: I am being facetious, of course, when I speak of "unnatural" water. What I mean is water that has been treated in a way to remove some or all of its harmful properties. The two forms we usually find are deionized water (sometimes called demineralized water) and steam-distilled water.

Deionizing water is a process using electrons to remove lead, cadmium, calcium, barium, magnesium, nitrates, and some forms of radium. Steam-distilled water has undergone vaporization. When the water is boiled, it turns to steam, leaving behind almost all bacteria and viruses. The steam itself passes through a condensing chamber, where it is cooled and becomes water once again.

Steam-distilled water has one other benefit. When you drink it, it leaches the inorganic minerals (sodium, potassium, etc.) from the body. These are minerals that have been rejected by cells and tissues but can cause harm if they remain in the body. The leaching process is a good thing!

What to Drink

I've studied many processes and different products for cleaning water as well as many different kinds of bottled water. In the course of this work, I had the unpleasant experience of discovering that a local supplier of spring water that seemed excellent was, in fact, bottling tap water and then mislabeling it.

Some home filtration systems do an effective job, but their cost is extremely high. My recommendation is that you buy steam-distilled water for all drinking and cooking needs, leaving the tap water for bathing and for washing clothes. It is the least expensive way to avoid the problems we face as our society periodically threatens the safety of our water.

TIPS FOR WATER AS A NATURAL REMEDY

1. Always consider your intake of distilled water to be separate from other beverages. Many liquids are diuretics; they cause you to lose water through urination. Caffeine is a diuretic, alcohol another. If you drink coffee, tea, or hot chocolate, you may be increasing your need for water, since you'll have more frequent urination. (Distilled water is the ideal, but use tap or other drinking water if you must.)

2. Cold water rehydrates more quickly than warm water. There was a time when athletic coaches thought there was something dangerous about cold water, so the football team's water boy would carry a bucket of water that was the same temperature as the air. Now we know that coldness causes the water to be absorbed faster and

utilized more efficiently. This phenomenon affects many creatures, which is why veterinarians tell you that cats need water that's cool to cold and may shun water that's too warm to quench their thirst.

3. Consider your minimum water intake to be eight eight-ounce glasses, but increase this to eight ounces per hour when you have a cold or other respiratory ailment.

4. Thirst is an indication of the loss of at least two cups of water. Until that point, you may not have the sensation of thirst. Still, you should be drinking water before you feel thirsty, especially when you're in hot, dry areas where the time between noticeable thirst and serious dehydration is extremely short.

5. Drink water throughout the day. If you have to, carry a water bottle with you. Remember, if you need to drive a long distance, you can put a chilled bottle in an insulated beverage cooler in your car.

6. Your body loses water when you sleep, so taking a long drink before you go to bed and another when you wake is an excellent idea, especially as you age. Keep in mind that starting your morning with coffee or tea will only cause you to lose more water.

7. The loss of water through perspiration is extensive. You perspire, you know, for several reasons, not just deliberately engaging in an exercise program. Sitting in the hot sun can cause severe fluid loss. You also lose moisture from normal physical activities such as carrying heavy

loads, climbing stairs, and taking a walk. You'll probably benefit from additional cups of water under such circumstances.

8. Locate a convenient source of water in your office, school, or wherever you spend your time. Then take regular water breaks.

9. Take regular water breaks while you're exercising. Don't wait until you're finished. The breaks for water will not harm your exercise routine, as some trainers once suspected.

AIR

The third natural remedy—actually a group of treatments known as bio-oxidative therapies—is still in an experimental phase in the United States. Various forms of the therapies have been successfully used in Europe for decades and they have also been tried on an experimental basis in this country. As of now, the outcome of some of these therapies has been so promising in treating diseases that have resisted other cures—cancer, AIDS, and some immune-system disorders—that I think it essential for you to know about them. You will find at the end of this chapter the addresses of three clearinghouses for information so that you can discuss the methods with your physician if the need arises or if you wish to learn more about them.

Bio-oxidative therapies revolve around two well-known products: ozone and hydrogen peroxide. Ozone is a form of oxygen containing extra electrons, which make it simultaneously deadly and a powerful tool in fighting disease.

Ozone, a pale blue gas, has three atoms of oxygen in every

molecule instead of the two atoms that constitute oxygen. It is best known as the shield against the sun's harmful ultraviolet light that lies 50,000 to 100,000 feet above the earth's surface.

The full importance of this shield was discovered only after human ignorance created chlorofluorocarbons (CFCs) for use in refrigerants and propellants. For years, many air conditioners, refrigerators, freezers, and aerosol spray cans used CFCs, which were released into the atmosphere, and over time, eroded the ozone layer, raising the risk of skin cancer and other immune-system disorders. Now all the nations of the world are working to eliminate the use of CFCs in the hope of saving the ozone layer. But ozone is more than just a gas that envelops the earth.

Ozone is the natural enemy of viruses and bacteria. The fact that it seems to have no harmful effect on humans and animals when it's used to treat our drinking water has led many communities to switch from chlorination and related treatment methods. Instead of relying on those often ineffective and dangerous chemical additives, they arrange to have ozone added to oxygen, then bubbled through the water they use for drinking. In this way, the viruses and bacteria are killed, and the microorganisms that give some water a bad taste or odd odor are neutralized.

Ozone also has numerous disinfectant and medicinal uses. For instance, every time you drink a bottled beverage, there's a chance that the inside of the container was disinfected by ozone. It is also used on sewage, oxidating the compounds so that they are odor free. It kills viruses in the bloodstream, improves blood circulation, and is helpful in treating everything from glaucoma and hepatitis to AIDS. These medical uses are still considered experimental in the United States, however, despite their regular application in Europe.

Hydrogen peroxide, a colorless liquid formed by ozone moving through water, is found in trace amounts in rain and snow, and, in somewhat larger quantities, in many fruits and vegetables. Tomatoes, apples, watermelons, oranges, and cabbage are among the natural sources of hydrogen peroxide that you probably consume.

Within the human body, hydrogen peroxide acts as an oxygenator, helping to deliver oxygen to the blood, organs, and tissues. It may also enhance our ability to utilize effectively the air we breathe.

Like ozone, hydrogen peroxide has been used to get rid of harmful bacteria and microorganisms. Farmers add it to the drinking water of farm animals; it apparently heightens both the volume and butterfat quantity of cow's milk. It also destroys the bacteria in the bulk storage containers used for the milk. Adding hydrogen peroxide to your own drinking water is discussed on page 80; at this time, it is an extremely controversial treatment, and caution is necessary.

Medical uses, though experimental, are extremely promising. For example, hydrogen peroxide has been used to enhance the oxygen reaching the heart of a patient who has suffered a heart attack. It is known to decrease the plaque buildup in arteries, thus keeping them clear. And it is capable of expanding blood vessels in all organs, including the brain. This can lead to a marked reduction or the elimination of your risk of stroke and other types of brain damage that once seemed a "natural" part of deterioration through aging. In the lungs, hydrogen peroxide stimulates the blood flow, increasing oxygenation, and helps to remove foreign matter and damaged tissue. However, there remain questions and controversy, so caution is in order when considering hydrogen peroxide use in water. I believe we may find this therapy to be dangerous for most people.

The list of its potential benefits seems endless. The more we learn about both ozone and hydrogen peroxide, the more exciting appears the future of this form of therapy. I cannot, however, stress enough that it is still experimental and that caution is required. It must also be noted that hydrogen peroxide produced within the body acts as a dangerous free radical, which means that it could turn out to be both a good and a bad guy.

BIO-OXIDATIVE THERAPY

The basic concept behind the use of both ozone and hydrogen peroxide in what are commonly called bio-oxidative therapies is a sound one. Certain disease-causing bacteria thrive where there is little or no oxygen; these bacteria are anaerobic. In fact, for more than thirty years we have known that anaerobic cells provide an environment that is hospitable to cancer.

We also know that when you expand the volume of oxygen reaching the cells, then parasites, germs, fungi, and diseased tissue are destroyed. More important, the healthy cells are revitalized.

Compare the use of these natural substances—which have few or no side effects when used correctly—with medications. Pharmaceuticals are foreign substances that can harm the body. Aggressive treatment for a serious disease like cancer calls for both chemotherapy and radiation therapy, each of which causes great trauma to the body. Nausea, hair loss, weight loss, and other problems accompany such treatments. As we saw in the example of the heartworm medicine, a therapy given incorrectly can kill. The hope, of course, is that the cancer will be destroyed before the "cure" causes greater damage.

We look forward to the day when bio-oxidation therapies that have been thoroughly tested in countries with reputable medical systems will be available to everyone who can benefit from them. Those therapies will be rigorously tested in the United States so that they can be adopted or modified for treatment. Certainly, the use of ozone and hydrogen peroxide seems destined to be a part of the future of medical professionals.

CURRENT THERAPIES

Please remember that current therapies are *not* medical quackery. These therapies, though little reported, have been used in other countries for many years, and the available international literature has impressed me with the facts about their safety (except as noted) and quality. In fact, I would guess that if ozone and hydrogen peroxide were pharmaceuticals, they'd be widely used right now.

The resistance to testing nonpharmaceutical therapies is a reality of the American medical system. Medical research costs money, often a lot of money. Although conducting research is a highly esteemed enterprise, hospitals and university medical schools have limited funds to offer research scientists. Just as some universities talk of "publish or perish" in the arts, a similar situation exists in medicine. The greatest respect, and often the best jobs, go to those physicians, biochemists, and other research scientists who bring in massive grants to fund their projects. The grants pay for laboratories, expensive equipment, and the salaries of graduate students. They help underwrite hospital costs. And they make the undergraduate and graduate programs more desirable.

The trouble is that research grants are most readily available from pharmaceutical companies, because it is often smarter for a business to give several million dollars to a researcher working in a university lab than to build additional facilities of its own. Providing the research money also ensures that diverse groups of patients can be tested with a given drug. For example, grants can be given to researchers in different parts of the country where the test subjects will come from various races, age groups, and ethnic backgrounds.

There is little altruism behind this. The pharmaceutical companies are not solely concerned with doing good, nor are they deeply interested in funding research on wellness—the prevention of disease and the ravages of age. And they certainly do not want to pay for research in fields from which they will not benefit.

Consequently, any researcher who wants to experiment with bio-oxidative therapies has only limited access to funds. Sometimes there are contributions from wealthy people who suffer from one disease or another and are aware of the potential of these alternative therapies. Sometimes research grants are available from endowments not connected with drug manufacturers. And sometimes researchers work out of pocket, earning their living through the practice of medicine, or teaching, and then paying for their experimentation as best they can. Thus, use and standardization of these practices have been slow to happen in the United States, but bio-oxidative therapies show much promise. It is hoped that many of the treatments discussed below may soon become as commonplace here as they are in other parts of the world like Europe and Asia. Refer to Appendix A for more information on these therapies.

1. *Intramuscular Injection:* This is a direct injection of an ozone-oxygen mixture into a large muscle mass, usually the buttocks, to treat allergies, cancer (as an adjunct to other therapies), and some inflammatory ailments.

2. *Rectal Insufflation:* This unpleasant-sounding therapy has so far been proven safe and effective for a variety of such health problems as cancer and AIDS. It is also simple enough so that some people have learned to deliver the ozone to themselves.

The technique involves taking between 100 and 800 milliliters of an oxygen-ozone mixture and sending it into the rectum by means of an apparatus like an enema tube, where it is absorbed through the intestines. The treatment takes no more than two minutes, and works for up to twenty minutes, long enough to bring about a major change, according to published reports. Improvements are noted for ulcerative colitis, some types of cancer, HIV-related problems, and others.

3. *Ozone Bagging:* This odd-sounding technique involves a bag filled with a mixture of ozone and oxygen being placed on the surface of the skin so that it completely encases the problem area—a severe burn, an ulcer, a fungal infection. There is, as well, an experimental AIDS technique involving a bag that encases the entire body *except* the head. The ozone-oxygen mixture is absorbed through the pores and works to heal the entire body. The use in other countries has so far yielded positive results, at least with the specific spot problems. The AIDS experimentation is still too new to present adequate statistics.

4. *Fractionalization:* Technically called autohomologous immunotherapy (AHT), this technique calls for the addition of ozone to the blood and urine. A patient suffering from one of a variety of problems, like rheumatoid arthritis,

cancer, asthma, premature aging, allergies, or a chronic infection, has quantities of blood and urine taken by the doctor. In the laboratory these are fractionalized—broken down biochemically on a cellular and liquid level. Then, the fractionalized blood is processed with ozone and other biochemicals and finally returned to the patient in whatever form is appropriate—through an inhalant, by injection, or with drops. As odd as this sounds, it is one of those therapies that seem ultimately headed to the United States because of their success.

5. *Ozone and Oil:* Olive oil—sometimes sunflower oil—is treated in a laboratory with ozone, and the resulting liquid is bottled for direct application to the skin. It is used in some hospitals for everything from acne to bedsores to leg ulcers. Its potential for at-home use is excellent.

6. *Intra-Articular Injection:* This process has the ozone bubbled through water and the resulting liquid injected between the joints. It is used in hospitals for arthritis and similar problems.

7. *Ozonated Water:* This is actually a variation of the preceding method. The liquid resulting from the ozone bubbled through the water is used as a cleansing wash for wounds, skin infections, and burns. Dentists use it in connection with surgical procedures, and some doctors use it for intestinal disorders.

8. *Autohemotherapy:* In this process, a quantity of blood is removed from the patient, treated with ozone and oxygen, then injected into a muscle or vein. For a muscle, the pro-

cedure is called minor autohemotherapy, in which no more than 10 milliliters of the patient's blood is used. For intravenous use, the technique is called major auto-hemotherapy, requiring the initial removal of as much as 100 milliliters of blood.

DANGEROUS THERAPIES

1. *Injection into Veins or Arteries:* This rarely used technique involves the slow injection of the oxygen-ozone mixture into a vein or artery. The doctor must take every precau-tion, when using the syringe, to go neither too slowly nor too rapidly. A slip either way poses a danger to the patient that outweighs the probability of improving the circula-tion of the arterial blood. Although this method is still practiced, the risks call it into question.

2. *Ozone Inhalation:* There are commercial air purifiers that send small amounts of ozone into the air to improve health—or so the advertisements claim. The problem is that any inhalation of ozone is dangerous. You could cause yourself life-threatening emphysema, among other problems, if you make any error. As with ozone bagging, even a minute quantity of ozone, though harmless within the bagged area, can be dangerous if it leaks into the air and is inhaled.

HYDROGEN PEROXIDE THERAPIES

1. *Bathing:* For this treatment, a pint of 35 percent food-grade hydrogen peroxide is added to the bathwater, and the patient lies in the water for at least twenty minutes,

allowing the diluted hydrogen peroxide to be absorbed through the skin. The method has been studied only anecdotally, but patients suffering from certain types of infections, rashes, and stiffness of the joints have said they gained relief. While its benefits are still unproven, the method is probably harmless.

2. *Intravenous Infusion:* This involves the careful preparation of 30 percent reagent hydrogen peroxide and sterile distilled water, which is made into a stock solution that is filtered and sterilized. A specific quantity of the solution is added to a liquid that is dripped intravenously into the patient over one to three hours. Treatments can range from one a week to one a day, depending on the problem and its severity. Because this is a controlled treatment whose results are known and whose side effects are minor, it is preferred by many physicians.

3. *Hydrogen Peroxide Injection:* A solution containing 0.03 percent hydrogen peroxide is injected into the joints to treat such inflammatory ailments as arthritis. It is intended to ease soft tissue problems.

USE EXTREME CAUTION

1. *Oral Ingestion:* Drops of 35 percent hydrogen peroxide are added to a glass of distilled water, which is then drunk. If this mixture is taken two or three times a day, it can relieve arthritis and serve as an appropriate adjunct to the treatment of several other illnesses, including cancer and heart disease. Note that only distilled water should be

used, because other forms of water may contain iron, a substance that reacts adversely to the hydrogen peroxide. Some physicians feel that extreme caution is necessary with oral ingestion. They believe that the body's fatty acids may cause some of the hydrogen peroxide to change into free radicals, leaving a destructive wake in the body. They recommend that all oral ingestion be avoided. I agree.

ADDITIONAL INFORMATION

Since bio-oxidation therapy remains controversial and unproven in the United States, you may want to keep track of the latest developments in the field. I include the following information because I believe that one or more of these therapies will soon be part of accepted medicine. These are some of the organizations keeping track of legitimate studies and current therapies:

ECHO (Ecumenical Catholic Help Organization), P.O. Box 126, Delano, MN 55328. A quarterly newsletter is published in Florida. The address is ECHO Newsletter, 9845 N.E. 2nd Avenue, Miami, FL 33138.

International Bio-Oxidative Medicine Foundation (IBOMF), P.O. Box 891954, Oklahoma City, OK 73109.

The International Ozone Association, Inc., Pan American Group, 31 Strawberry Hill Avenue, Stamford, CT 06902.

Chapter Three

A Brief Word About the Use of
NATURAL REMEDIES
AND YOUR BODY

AS YOU READ the next few chapters, you may think I've dropped the subject of natural remedies, because I'll be discussing the supplements I want you to use when you're feeling well. You may have the impression that a natural remedy is like a pharmaceutical—a reactive strike in the battle against ill health—and to a degree you're right. Everything discussed will have a specific benefit for one problem or another. Sometimes the natural remedy is to be used in conjunction with another form of therapy; sometimes it is to be used alone. But if you wish to think of natural remedies solely as God's reactive medicine, you may miss the important information in this book.

American society believes in sickness far more than in wellness. We somehow expect disease and disability to be a driving force in all that we do. You don't believe me? Think about your job.

Either before you took your job or at some point after you'd been at it for a while, you started thinking about benefits, like vacation time. It's minor but important, of course. We all want time away from the job; we all like the idea of being paid to stay home or travel. And if the vacation arrangements aren't great, you'll probably stay awhile and then consider going elsewhere.

Retirement issues are of interest, too. Is there a retirement plan? When do you become vested? What are your options? Again, if it's not all to your liking, you may stay a while and then look for a different place, where you can do the same sort of work but have a better retirement program to look forward to.

Finally, there are health benefits. Now I suspect I have your attention. Do you have an HMO or a PPO? Do you have full family coverage? Do you have dental care? Eye care? Pregnancy benefits? I'll bet that your health care coverage is not only something you know more about than your retirement plan; I'll bet it's one of your prime considerations for staying with your job.

Medical benefits are an obsession with job seekers and dissatisfied job holders. They are the reason some people stay in a boring, dead-end job. They're the first concern of the entrepreneur and the "downsized" employee. Depending on your age, you may be worried about pregnancy or menopause, heart disease or cancer, hospital emergency services for children, arthritis, cataracts . . . The list goes on and on. Name your fears based on personal experience, the experience of friends, or the genetic predispositions of your family, and you'll find your reason for clinging to a dull job in order to assure yourself of coverage. Even if your family's history is one of good health and long life, the comments of friends probably make you so nervous that you believe you'll need what the previous generations didn't need. And if you do leave your job, by choice or otherwise, you're likely to worry yourself sick about how you're going to get care if disaster strikes.

Natural remedies require you to think differently. As you have seen, in many instances pharmaceuticals do nothing more than duplicate, unnaturally, the effects of plants found in different parts of the world. Natural remedies, however, respond to the body's problems. Natural remedies can prevent illness, or delay its arrival. And if you do get sick, they can make the illness less severe and debilitating than would otherwise be the case.

In Chapter 4, you'll learn about cereal grasses and extracts of young green barley leaves that are so nutritious, they constitute what might be called the perfect food. They've been used successfully to treat the devastation of Alzheimer's disease and the inflammatory problems of arthritis, among other problems. But more important, their regular use, and the use of other natural remedies, will prevent illness. Many of the remedies slow the distressing effects of aging, as melatonin does. And most of them strengthen the immune system in a manner that prevents disease.

The problem with attempting to quantify the benefits of natural remedies is that the data are largely personal and anecdotal. There have been, and continue to be, studies of these remedies that involve the same treatment modalities and double-blind studies used for pharmaceuticals. I have drawn heavily on such information so that what I provide you with is accurate, up to date, and covers all known problems.

But anecdotal evidence is something that cannot be discounted with any product—pharmaceutical or natural—that promotes wellness. This is an intensely personal situation based on individual body chemistry, and that is the problem of applying the scientific method.

For example, a friend of mine who is a writer regularly travels to other cities by air. He either gets little sleep because of his assignments, or sleep that comes in snatches between his interviews of people like police officers, who work on different shifts. Because he is hypoglycemic, his body suffers from jet lag and from the pressure changes within the jetliners, a problem that also afflicts diabetics and users of alcohol.

For years my friend would return home exhausted and weak. He'd get a sore throat, a runny nose, a headache, and if flu was making its rounds, his body would embrace it with a vengeance. If his kids got sick, he'd catch whatever they brought home.

Then he began to experiment with natural remedies as preventive measures. He used melatonin, for example, both to handle sleep and to deal better with the stress caused by having to sleep in three- and four-hour bits. He took St. John's wort, because, in the past, his exhaustion had led to mood changes and to serious depression that lasted two, three, or four weeks, sometimes longer. He took saw palmetto, because there was a history of prostate troubles in his family. And he began using other products, some as familiar as vitamin C and B complex vitamins. He sometimes found the items in discount stores. The expenses upped his budget by only a few dollars a month, less than he and his wife spent lunching out together every few weeks.

Within a matter of days, my friend noticed a change in his health. If he became tired because of his work, was unable to eat at appropriate times, he did *not* degenerate into depression, as he would have during the preceding twenty years. He could travel, experience jet lag and a degree of sleep deprivation, and then return and find that getting extra rest each day was all he needed. There were no colds. There was no influenza. His body stopped acting like a basket for every germ his children brought home from school or day care. His productivity rose. His mood leveled off in a healthy manner. And his health was better than it had been in years.

His wife made similar changes, choosing natural remedies based on her particular needs. She too found that wellness was her normal situation. In fact, she has recently left a job she hated, a job with great stress that she'd kept only because of the health care benefits. As she put it, "The job was causing me to need the benefits. My changes in diet and exercise patterns have so improved my health that I've stopped thinking of sickness as inevitable. I know I should have some kind of policy; anyone can be injured in an accident and go through an expensive recovery. But for the price of a few supplements, I was able to leave the work I hated and become healthier at the same time. My new job really brings me satisfaction, not just the visits to the HMO."

I've known people whose early stages of cataracts went into remission once they started a natural remedy like melatonin. There is definite medical evidence of such remission, which in some cases lasted for a number of years. It was not the cataracts that prompted the people to take the melatonin; they were using it as a sleep aid. But their health improved in several ways. The remission of the cataracts, picked up by their ophthalmologists, was one of the first.

As always, of course, you must remember to take precautions. Once you start on the supplements, keep in mind that many medicines actually mimic them or react negatively with the changes that they cause in body chemistry. When people began trying the antidepressant herb St. John's wort, for instance, without stopping the use of drugs like Prozac, they overdosed. They thought they could wean themselves off the medicine while using the supplement, but that brought trouble.

Garlic, which we'll discuss in Chapter 5, has been known to

interact in a dangerous way with some pharmaceutical blood thinners, as have other natural remedies, like vitamin E.

When you start to use natural remedies as preventive measures, be certain to mention each one to both your doctor and your pharmacist. Understand that you're altering your body's physiology with natural medicines. So, although you are using the plants of creation, you have to remember that many of them are mimicked by pharmaceuticals, and can interact negatively with each other in the same way that pharmaceuticals, harmless when taken alone, can be dangerous when taken together. We know that this was the case when two different diet drugs were combined for "greater efficiency," only to have doctors discover the combination could be deadly.

Does this mean you should avoid certain natural remedies? Absolutely not. You can find information about their proper use in this book. But I want you to be aware that when you're doing the right thing for your body, when you're focusing on wellness instead of illness, you are still making changes in the body's delicate chemistry. Treat everything with respect, and do not mix natural remedies with pharmaceuticals unless you're under the close supervision of a doctor or other medical expert who understands fully the possible chemical interactions of the two remedies.

Chapter Four

GREEN FOODS

NO, THIS CHAPTER is not going to tell you to eat your spinach, your broccoli, and your asparagus, all of which are green, tasty, and nutritious. Instead, it's going to discuss some of the green foods you normally don't read of, green foods that can save your life. These are the cereal grasses, like wheat and barley. Although they are rarely mentioned as natural therapies, they remain among the most important preventives of both breast and prostate cancer. In fact, laboratory studies have shown that both prevention *and* treatment of such dreaded illnesses as prostate and breast cancer can be achieved through barley grass.

CHLOROPHYLL

If you or your children are fans of the Muppets, you may know the song "It's Not Easy Being Green." Kermit the frog sings the tune about racism, prejudice, and self-acceptance. But this song could also be sung about chlorophyll, the green liquid that is essential for health and is also potentially dangerous.

If you know the term "chlorophyll," chances are you learned it through the advertisements for toothpaste that were popular more than thirty years ago. Television commercials showed handsome young men and beautiful young women brushing their teeth with a toothpaste that boasted chlorophyll as one of its major ingredients. Then these great-looking people would go to work or engage in some form of recreation and smile at each other during a chance encounter. Suddenly, as though chlorophyll were Cupid's aphrodisiac, they were in love, soon to be partners for life. The toothpaste had cleaned their teeth, the chlorophyll had cleaned their breath, and this marvelous form of oral hygiene guaranteed that they would live happily ever after.

Not that the idea was an advertiser's fantasy. A decade earlier, the *Journal of the American Medical Association* discussed research indicating that chlorophyll derivatives held the promise of stopping internal body odors, a fact that would lead to more pleasant personal encounters. It was the first time that chlorophyll and romance had been linked, though the serious medical journal did not promote that link the way the toothpaste manufacturers did.

Romance is alive and well, but you don't hear much about chlorophyll today. Now different ingredients are hyped to sell toothpaste, mouthwash, and other oral hygiene products. For, although chlorophyll remains a powerful germicide, and an effective anti-inflammatory that protects the internal organs of people suffering from gastritis or peptic ulcers, it has been found to be unstable—a fact that makes it potentially dangerous.

Chlorophyll has been compared by some researchers with the human blood. They refer to chlorophyll as the "blood" of plants, and the analogy is quite appropriate when you consider the chemical composition of each. Hemoglobin (blood) and chlorophyll are indeed similar; just about the only difference is that hemoglobin contains iron bonded in its structure and chlorophyll contains magnesium.

The chlorophyll introduced as an additive to toothpaste and other products was not in its natural state, because natural chlorophyll, when heated, oxidized, or placed in an acidic environment, will break down to little more than green pigment, and lose its therapeutic value. Therefore, it was mixed with copper chlorophyllin sodium, a substance consisting of a copper ion bound to decomposed natural chlorophyll. It is stable, water soluble, and does not lose its color when exposed to sunlight. It also cannot be absorbed in the body except in amounts so minute as to have no effect whatever, an important health factor. This artificial chlorophyll is actually as deadly as natural chlorophyll becomes when oxidized. It creates a by-product called pheophorbide. Above a certain concentration, pheophorbide can be fatal. The creation of pheophorbide makes it imperative that chlorophyll used for human consumption in any form must not be oxidized.

Japan is one country that takes the problem of pheophorbide so seriously that it regulates the amount of pheophorbide-causing chlorophyll a product may have. The amount of pheophorbide is determined by the distance between the growing fields and the processing plant, the time lapse between harvesting and processing, and the method of processing, such as cooking or freeze-drying. There is also concern about an imbalance caused when acidic elements such as alcohol are added in the processing. Only when such matters are known, and when the pheophorbide has been measured, can you determine whether a chlorophyll supplement is safe. For the time being, you should not use chlorophyll as a supplement; you should obtain it indirectly through other foods. The ideal source, which will be discussed shortly, is barley grass. First, though, I want to tell you about a substance known as chlorella.

CHLORELLA

Chlorella is a single-cell alga with a large quantity of chlorophyll in its nucleus. Although very new information now indicates chlorella is unsafe, for many years it was considered one of the few edible algae, a cleanser of the bloodstream, and a source of numerous nutrients. And what nutrients they are!

Chlorella contains beta-carotene and all the B vitamins (including more B_{12} than liver). It contains vitamin E, several trace minerals, amino acids, carbohydrates, and proteins. And it is high in RNA and in DNA, and provides ultraviolet-light protection. Eating processed chlorella was long thought to be the equivalent of eating a complete meal, the protein alone ensuring the good health of those who need meat protein but cannot or choose not to eat it.

However . . .

One of Japan's leading medical researchers specializing in nutritional alternatives to pharmaceuticals is Yoshihide Hagiwara, M.D. For many years he headed a pharmaceutical research company that produced a broad range of medicines used throughout the world, including the United States. But there came a time when he found that some of these pharmaceuticals did little good for the patients, and some of them had side effects as unhealthy in their way as the illnesses they were supposed to heal. When he began experimenting with nutrition, analyzing the effectiveness of both little-known nutrients like cereal grasses and substances previously thought beneficial, he discovered that chlorella was in the latter category.

According to Dr. Hagiwara, chlorella, a hard-cell membrane that is difficult to digest, shows little or no sign of any genetic evolution that has taken place over the last three thousand years. He noted that when a food company devised a chlorella-rich yogurt as a health product, a large number of those who ate it became ill. That product and a similarly enriched beverage were removed from the market.

Dr. Hagiwara's conclusion was that chlorella, under the best of circumstances, is not as helpful as was once hoped. And under some circumstances, it is potentially harmful. This was why he too turned his focus to the cereal grasses.

CEREAL GRASSES

Long green cereal grasses are the early stages of barley, oats, rye, wheat, and other cereal plants. Unlike the grains they eventually become, though, the grasses have more in common with leafy green vegetables. In fact, a person with an allergy to wheat would probably have no problem eating wheat grass, the plant's earlier stage of development.

Earlier, I mentioned that our technologically advanced society has led us to deplete our foodstuffs of most of their nutritional value. This is the outgrowth of processing and preserving almost all that we eat, instead of ingesting it raw. Of all the preservation methods, freezing is the least destructive, yet it's recently been found that frozen food has lost many of the nutrients essential for health. This is one of the reasons that cereal grasses are so important. They supply nutrients that are lost through food processing.

Note: I am often criticized for sounding like an alarmist. I've heard people say that food can't be the problem I say it is. After all, the methods for preserving and shipping food have helped to alleviate hunger and to encourage the growth of cities where people can't grow their own food. They have, that is, contributed to the betterment of the world.

Yes, there's much truth to these claims. But what is not noted is that by "improving" the food we eat, we create problems that never existed. It's only since we've become an urban society and stopped living off the land that we've been plagued by immune-deficiency disorders, arteriosclerosis, hypertension, heart disease, atherosclerosis, and a dramatic rise in the incidence of cancer. We may be taller than we were in the past, but that doesn't mean we're stronger. We may indeed be endangering ourselves through improper diet.

BARLEY GRASS

While barley grass is not the single answer to our health problems, it is the most complete preventive medicine available. There's growing evidence that it helps in fighting such ailments as a dangerously low level of potassium in the blood (hypokalemia), heart problems, cancer, arthritis, and other inflammatory ailments. Its nutrient value serves to reduce or eliminate ailments caused by malnutrition, among the most widespread health problems of the population, especially among teenagers. (Malnutrition does not mean that you're hungry. You may even be eating in such quantities as to become obese. But volume of food, even type of food, is no guarantee of nutritive value.)

Barley could be considered one of the ultimate gifts of God. Anyone who has read the Old Testament knows of the journey of Moses and the Hebrew people to the Promised Land. The Book of Deuteronomy describes that land as having been worth the forty years of wandering in the desert. Deuteronomy 8:7–8 reads, in part: "For the Lord your God is bringing you into a good land, a land with flowing streams, with springs and underground waters welling up in valleys and hills, a land of wheat and barley . . ." Biblical scholars believe that barley was the first crop planted on the Jericho Plain and harvested in March, with a second harvest in the highlands of Jerusalem, mentioned in the Book of Ruth. Both the Old and New Testaments show that the reaping and binding of the barley sheaves took place from Passover through Pentecost.

Throughout history, barley was sown after the heavy October rains. The plowman would dig the furrows in the softened earth, and the sower would drop in the barley seed. The ritual was so familiar that Jesus used it as an image in a parable, Matthew 13:3–8: "A sower went out to sow. And as he sowed, some seeds fell on the path, and the birds came and ate them up. Other seeds fell on rocky ground, where they did not have much soil, and they sprang up quickly, since they had no depth of soil. But when the sun rose, they were scorched; and since they had no root, they withered away. Other seeds fell among thorns, and the thorns grew up and choked them. Other seeds fell on good soil and brought forth grain, some a hundredfold, some sixty, some thirty."

Barley was so important to health that farmers did not harvest all of it from their fields. Gleanings were left along the edge so that the poor would be able to make the nutritious bread they needed for good health.

The beneficial qualities of barley bread are supported by the story in John 6:1–14, telling of Jesus feeding the five thousand people who had come to hear him speak shortly before Passover. When Jesus asked how to get food for those who had gathered, Andrew, the brother of Simon Peter, said, "There is a

boy here who has five barley loaves and two fish. B
they among so many people?" Jesus had this peasan
tributed among the people, and "from the fragments or tne nve
barley loaves, left by those who had eaten, they filled twelve
baskets."

The miracle in the Bible was that Jesus fed five thousand
with five barley loaves and two fish. The miracle for us is the
barley itself, and the benefits that the green barley leaves continue to offer us. Today, many knowledgeable people consume
the juice of the green barley leaves, often in the form of a tablet
or powder to be mixed with water. It is sold as Green Magma
and as Green Barley Essence. The leaves, or their powdered
form, contain calcium, chlorophyll, copper, magnesium, manganese, organic iron, phosphorus, potassium, zinc, and the enzyme superoxide dismutase.

And that is just what we know for certain! We continue to
discover previously unknown health benefits all the time. There
is, for example, an antioxidant that inhibits lipid peroxidation.
This is a technical way of saying that it fights the buildup of
hydrogen peroxide in fat cells and tissues, where it can be extremely destructive. This antioxidant, with the tongue-twisting
name of 2-0-Glycosyl Isovitexin, or 2-0-GIV, is one of the most
potent you can take, and it is found in barley leaves. Researchers dealing with arthritis and other inflammatory diseases are
also finding that patients can gain measurable and quick relief
by consuming green barley, as do people with pancreatitis and
disorders of the colon, duodenum, and stomach.

Green barley enzymes neutralize cancer-causing substances
like tobacco tar, and the green barley extract has been found, in
laboratory tests, to destroy prostate cancer cells. It improves the
circulatory system and strengthens the immune system—and

this is just what we know now! Green barley research is in its infancy, so we may soon learn of even more benefits to be obtained from it.

As you can see, it is surely fair to believe that green barley may be nature's one-stop answer to a huge number of health problems and illnesses plaguing people all over the world.

PHYTOCHEMICALS

You might think that if you maintain a proper diet, you would have no reason to take a supplement. After all, if whole foods are flash-frozen or prepared in some manner that preserves them soon after they've been harvested, why do we need to worry about these grains and grasses? This seems especially true for people who try to do everything "right," like using one of the popular home breadmakers and eating organically grown vegetables.

This logic is excellent, but recently scientists have identified a specific group of natural chemicals that deteriorate when subjected to processing. These are the phytochemicals, that is, plant chemicals like carotenoids, flavonoids, phenolic acids, and tocopherols—all excellent antioxidants. The problems caused by the loss of these chemicals can be minimized if you supplement your diet with green grasses and by eating more fruits and vegetables.

ALFALFA TABLETS

If you suffer from arthritis, you may already know about alfalfa tablets, because more and more physicians have joined knowledgeable health food store owners in recommending them. They contain the minerals necessary for bone formation and were the first green food supplements to come on the market. They've long been known to have high mineral content. The fact that their roots grow ten to twenty feet into the earth is also important, since they are less likely to be affected by the pollutants and hazards that damage the shallow roots of other plants.

SUPPLEMENT USE

If you're working with a doctor or nutritionist, he or she may already have recommended the amount of green barley essence you should consume. Research is still so new that most experts recommend one or two glasses a day, though some people drink a single glass a day, much the way you might take a multiple vitamin. Other people use it as a specific response to a problem like gastritis; they take one or two glasses a day only while they experience the problem—a single day or several weeks.

Among the tasks at which green barley is most effective is the balancing of acidic and alkaline foods. The American diet is centered on meat, and meat is an acidic food. Because we eat few alkaline foods, such as vegetables, our body chemistry is often out of balance. An out-of-balance chemistry drastically lowers the immune system and allows illness to take hold.

Cells use minerals to maintain the acid-alkaline balance. They take in and give off minerals as needed. And enzymes, also essential for health, require minerals that are dissolved as ions in cell fluids to maintain proper metabolism.

Potassium is one of the most critical minerals, because it has a high ionizing effect. It is used for energy metabolism; if it drops, the osmotic pressure of the cell membrane is adversely affected.

Green barley provides stability, the reason it is so important. It is rich in potassium, B-complex vitamins, and other essential nutrients. We may not be able to recommend a specific amount beyond what you'll find suggested on the container, but we know enough about green barley to praise it as one of nature's most perfect foods.

Chapter Five

GARLIC, GINSENG, AND *GINKGO BILOBA*

No one is neutral about garlic, just as no one is neutral about skunks. Some people love the look of a skunk's soft, furry body, its quizzical face, its seemingly gentle demeanor. Others bluntly say that a skunk stinks, and they want nothing to do with it.

And then there's garlic. Some cuisines seem to start with garlic, the other ingredients, like tomatoes, herbs, and shellfish, serving as mere afterthoughts. There are gourmets, bon vivants, and, if truth be told, gluttons who all speak of garlic the way wine connoisseurs speak of their favorite vintage and cheese lovers talk of the subtle distinctions in flavor of one variety over another.

The garlic haters, on the other hand, say it smells terrible. They can't stand the way it comes out on the breath, the way the odor seems to ooze through the pores of the eater. They even joke that garlic is an excellent method of birth control; if one lover eats garlic, the other will maintain a distance of at least ten feet. For some people, garlic is even mildly toxic, upsetting their stomachs.

Garlic and alcohol are substances that are not metabolized.

They are absorbed through the stomach lining, which is why they leave the telltale odor. And it's why some people are sick to the stomach after ingesting them.

Fortunately, there is an aged garlic product that is detoxified and thus deodorized. Just as deodorized skunks make great house pets, so the more sociable garlic, with slightly altered chemistry and sold under the name Kyolic, can be used by people who can't eat ordinary garlic. In fact, a number of studies indicate that Kyolic may be more effective than raw garlic when it comes to boosting the body's immune system.

Why is garlic, in its original form or as the extract of the aged vegetable, good for you? Garlic contains germanium and selenium, which are sulfur-containing antioxidants that boost the immune system. In the study mentioned, conducted by Dr. Tariq Abdullah, Kyolic killed 20 percent more of the tumor cells in laboratory cultures than did raw garlic. And raw garlic is by itself one of the most potent boosters of your natural killer cells.

Kyolic has also been found more beneficial for hypoglycemics—people with low blood sugar levels—than raw garlic. The latter lowers the blood sugar level, unfortunately, but Kyolic stabilizes it. The aging process that creates Kyolic produces a supplement whose benefits I find stronger than those of raw garlic.

As enthusiastic as I am about barley grass, if someone were to ask me which single supplement he or she should use, I would recommend Kyolic garlic. It is among the oldest and most versatile of the documented natural remedies. When Hippocrates, the father of diagnostic medicine, was busy noting which treatments worked for the Greek people he treated, he listed garlic. A total of twenty-two ancient Egyptian remedies were found to use garlic, as noted in the Ebers Papyrus dating from the sixteenth century B.C.E. Garlic was a tool against the plague when it struck Marseilles in the 1770s. Albert Schweitzer found that, when he ran out of pharmaceutical supplies in his African mission, garlic successfully stopped dysentery. Louis Pasteur discovered that garlic had antibacterial properties. The Vikings would not go on long sea voyages without garlic. And, of course, as we know from fiction, garlic is an excellent defense against vampires.

Garlic was so valuable to the ancients that quantities of garlic, along with onions, were used to sustain the health of the men who built the Pyramids of Egypt. And today garlic has been beneficial in the treatment of such respiratory illnesses as bronchitis and asthma. It has been used to treat stomach ulcers and tuberculosis. And it has antifungal qualities that have made it valuable in treating athlete's foot.

It is rare that a natural remedy like garlic should appear so prominently in early medical literature. Barley, we know, is mentioned in the Bible, but in the medical knowledge that has been passed down through the centuries, garlic comes up repeatedly. Garlic can surely be considered one of the oldest medicines human beings have been able to understand and utilize, a natural remedy respected today, as it was in ancient times.

Garlic's value for your heart is well known. First, it contains properties for fighting "bad" cholesterol. We know now that high-density lipoprotein (HDL) cholesterol is not dangerous, but low-density lipoprotein (LDL) certainly is, because it can be oxidized by dangerous free radicals. Oxidized LDL is an enemy of the white blood cells, which become enlarged as "foam cells," and ultimately are deposited on the arterial walls in the form of plaque. The lumen, the open space of the artery, becomes more and more narrow until it is completely clogged.

HDL works in a more positive fashion. It is thicker than

LDL and acts a little like an older sibling assigned to keep the younger one out of trouble. HDL, in a way, takes the LDL by the scruff of the neck and escorts it to the liver, where it is broken down and removed from the body. LDL behaves itself only if it has not been oxidized. And it is the antioxidant quality of garlic that so diminishes the free radical damage to the cholesterol that LDL doesn't need its sibling HDL to hang around. It can be safely removed by itself. The result is that the garlic reduces the start and the progression of arteriosclerosis.

Heart patients, therefore, are especially blessed by garlic, but it is important to check with your doctor before adding garlic to your regimen, because there are pharmaceuticals that match its chemical properties. This is especially the case with popular blood thinners. In fact, Germany licenses garlic supplements as drugs for the treatment of arteriosclerosis.

In the 1920s, the world was introduced to one of the most valuable yet dangerous drugs ever created. This was aspirin, and 25 percent of all people will, at some point, have a serious, perhaps life-threatening reaction to it. Even more important, some children may develop Reye's syndrome from aspirin because their body chemistry is not sufficiently stable. Yet despite the risks, most emergency medical physicians and heart experts say that at the first sign of heart attack, you should take an aspirin and then call 911, because aspirin thins the blood, and this can delay or prevent a heart attack.

Garlic is natural aspirin, not because it contains salicylic acid, which was first identified in willow bark tea as a substance to ease headaches and reduce joint inflammation, but because it can help to prevent red blood cells from clumping together. Other qualities of garlic, so different from aspirin that they present no risk, dissolve clots and lengthen clotting time. This natural thinning of the blood helps every aspect of blood flow within your body. It is the safest source of prevention of heart attacks and strokes. Keeping that aspirin bottle tucked in with emergency medical supplies is still a good idea, but the regular consumption of Kyolic will almost certainly preclude the need for more drastic measures.

There are two common types of family illnesses, the first of them related to lifestyle. We physicians see this most clearly in conditions like diabetes. There are many causes of diabetes, but in some families it is the result of poor diet and lack of exercise. In these cases, the family looks upon children who gorge themselves as "healthy eaters." By this I don't mean they eat a wide range of nutritious foods in appropriate quantities. I mean that they eat heavily, sometimes disproportionately consuming desserts and high-sugar snacks.

The reasons for this are manifold. Children of Holocaust survivors frequently were seriously overweight by the time they reached their teens in the 1960s. Why? Because the parents, who had known terrible physical deprivation, unconsciously equated excess with freedom.

Another example is a friend who was taught that sitting down with a container of milk and a carton of cookies was good. His mother, who had been raised at a time when nutrition "experts" believed that sugar represented "empty calories"—it did nothing to benefit you, but it certainly wouldn't hurt you—had no idea that sugar robbed the body of B-complex vitamins and caused many serious difficulties. One of the worst was a severe immune deficiency.

There was yet another factor in his story. For his first six years, he lived in a two-family house where his mother was not happy. She projected her unhappiness onto her children, and was certain her little boy was sad because he didn't have his own yard. His being skinny, she decided, was proof of his misery.

When the family moved to their own house with their own yard, my friend, then seven, was encouraged to overindulge. "Filling out" was a sign that he was happy. The fact that he became fat was not something she considered. Only when he became an adult and developed hypoglycemia did he understand that his overeating had been a misguided attempt by his mother to make him happy.

We know that garlic provides a benefit for the cardiovascular system. Perhaps you or someone you know has a little difficulty in walking. It doesn't seem serious, but maybe it's reached the point where you just don't want to walk any more than you have to. You find that your legs feel weak, or you have a certain amount of leg pain. And when you stop walking to pause for a rest or sit down, the discomfort goes away.

That discomfort is caused by poor blood circulation in your legs. The technical term for the problem is intermittent claudication. Since it is known that garlic improves circulation to the body's peripheries, studies were conducted with patients experiencing this problem. The regular use of garlic lengthened the distance they could walk without weakness or discomfort. And as a side benefit, their cholesterol levels were lowered, and their blood pressure dropped to a healthy level.

Note: Genetic predisposition studies of the benefits of foods such as garlic are not and can never be scientifically proven. Researchers prefer double-blind studies in which several people with the same general body types and conditions are divided into two groups and given long-term treatment. One group is given the substance (food, supplement, or drug) under study, and the other group is given a placebo. The trouble is that to do such studies—and they would be ideal when twins are found in families predisposed to early death—is to assure that half the subjects will die. You have to "kill" 50 percent to prove your theory.

Instead, genetic-predisposition studies have to be done anecdotally in families whose backgrounds can be scientifically checked. One of my friends, for example, knows the diet, exercise, and death patterns of several generations on his father's side. No one lived more than fifty-six years until his father changed his diet and exercise pattern upon being diagnosed diabetic. (The others continued as always, if anything choosing to exercise less.) His father lived to be eighty-four, eventually dying from prostate cancer. My friend has avoided diabetes, and his children are being raised on diets with little sugar intake within active lifestyles, including long walks which they all find enjoyable, even those who are not athletically inclined.

What will we conclude from my friend, his father, and his children's lives? We will find anecdotal evidence that the family history will become just that—a curiosity of the past. He has avoided the "inevitable," as will his children after him if they remember the lessons of their youth.

This is what happens when garlic becomes part of the diet and supplement program of those with heart problems. In these cases, we know that individuals who, by all rights of family history, should be experiencing problems with their hearts are not having problems. They are doing better than their ancestors. In longer-term studies, they have outlived everyone simply by adding garlic in one form or another.

Are these individuals genetically unique? Possibly, but it is doubtful. Instead, it is safe to assume that the garlic made the difference. Yet this is not scientific methodology. It is just common sense, which, when it comes to the use of garlic to counter genetics, makes for good medicine.

Where scientific methods can be applied, as with antibacterial factors, garlic has been repeatedly proven safe and effective. Probably every woman and most men have heard of "yeast infection" (a.k.a. yeast syndrome or chronic candidiasis), a term defined mostly through symptoms. Blood tests or stool cultures can reveal the infection. But usually it is determined through a careful, complete physical history that reveals such problems as depression, irritability, vaginal yeast infections, frequent bladder infections, chronic fatigue, lack of energy, reduced sex drive, inability to concentrate, and other distresses. Any one of these is a concern; several in combination generally indicate the presence of chronic candidiasis.

Because yeast infections, along with fungus problems and viral infections, are not usually life-threatening, double-blind studies have been carried out on garlic as a treatment. The findings from these studies have repeatedly shown the value of garlic, in some cases used alone, and in others administered in combination with other natural therapeutics.

Note: Be certain not to self-medicate with garlic in response to the problems mentioned above. With candidiasis, for example, there may be several other concerns. You must eliminate from your diet alcohol, high-sugar foods, and other substances with a high-yeast or mold content. Your digestion must be improved. Detoxification of the liver must be pursued and the immune system strengthened. Then you must coordinate your efforts with your doctor's for continued treatment, because yeast infections can lie dormant and suddenly return if you fail to continue your care after the immediate flare-up.

Garlic is also excellent in the handling of body fat. This does not mean that you can eat garlic instead of getting exercise. You might be able to scare a vampire, but sloth, indolence, and overindulgence have no fear of garlic. Garlic, however, is acknowledged as one of the most effective means of reducing fat in conjunction with a healthy diet and exercise program.

This is not to say that you can eat all you want, using garlic as a magic pill. What you eat and how much you eat determine one source of fat, perhaps the most controllable source of fat in your body. The younger you are, the easier it is to burn the fat you take in through diet. As you get older, the ability to burn fat decreases. You may be as active at forty as you were at twenty, but you will find that a diet that left you with a flat stomach and slim hips in your youth is now forcing you to go to a larger size of clothing. This is natural and not unhealthy, but excess fat is never a good situation.

Note: Recent reports of long-term studies on body weight and health show that excess weight alone is not the danger it was once believed to be. The more excess fat you carry, the greater the stress on your body, but repeated dieting causes even greater stress. An important factor is your volume of exercise. An overweight person whose weight is stable, who is physically active, and who eats a healthy diet, including the appropriate supplements, will be far better off than the "hard body" whose diet and exercise habits are wrong. To be fat is not necessarily to be unhealthy. It is simply the most visible sign of a potentially dangerous condition that may manifest itself if you do not respect all the other factors that insure good health.

The fat we scold for clinging to our bodies as we age comes

from two sources. One fat stays there because our bodies fail to break it down and eliminate it. The other fat is made by our bodies, a process known as endogenous lipogenesis. Both may be products of our lifestyle as much as our age and eating habits.

For example, do you drink? I don't mean to excess. I mean a beer after work or some wine with dinner. Nothing to worry about. Nothing excessive.

What you probably don't realize is that the alcohol you consume interferes with the breakdown of dietary fats and stimulates endogenous lipogenesis. In other words, alcohol triggers the body's fat-producing mechanism and inhibits the body's ability to break down and eliminate fat.

Taking garlic is not an excuse to drink. I don't want to see you spending your happy hour sipping margaritas and downing quantities of Kyolic. However, garlic does slow or stop our body's production of fat by breaking down the lipids and enhancing the elimination of various by-products. Garlic also moves lipids from tissue to the bloodstream for eventual removal. Garlic can dramatically reduce the bad consequences of a multitude of dietary "sins." It truly is a good thing.

Perhaps one of the most promising findings of research on the use of garlic has come in the field of cancer. The Memorial Sloan-Kettering Cancer Center in New York has found that garlic inhibits the growth of cancer cells in the laboratory. And in a study of colon cancer conducted at the M. D. Anderson Hospital in Houston, Dr. Michael Wargovich determined that diallyl sulfide, a major component of garlic, reduced the growth of colon cancer in mice. A related experiment showed that diallyl sulfide may prevent cancer of the esophagus and help in preventing prostate cancer in some individuals.

The experiments have been thorough and the results encouraging. Garlic is gradually proving to be an effective treatment for cancer as well as a preventive, and is now being tried, in conjunction with other treatments, on immune-system disorders like AIDS. Laboratory results are consistently positive, and trials on humans show similar findings, though they are not yet far enough along for garlic to be stipulated as a treatment. However, as I said at the start of this chapter, if I had to take just one supplement for my health, it would be Kyolic garlic.

GINSENG

Ginseng, although it was used for centuries throughout parts of Asia, was one of the dirty little secrets of the Cold War. During the final years of tension between the United States and the Soviet Union, some military theorists posited that it would be wise to attack around four in the morning. From what you've learned about melatonin, you can understand the reasoning. That is the time of deepest sleep and least alertness. Of course, the commanders would be hard put to keep needed troops fully on the alert.

The basic idea was to have the attack be as much of a surprise to the attackers as those being attacked. This may sound crazy, but, as you know, when you're planning a surprise, it is important for as few people as possible to know about it beforehand. This prevents leaks. The military wanted to know what drugs could be stockpiled and administered to the troops to bring them instantly to peak alertness.

The complete list of drugs used for the experiments remains classified, though some are known. In the United States, for example, one was cocaine. It is a fast-acting stimulant, does not seem to inhibit performance in any way, and requires little enough per soldier so that packing an adequate quantity would not be a problem. That it was illegal was the only drawback, and caused great controversy at the time, although the drug was never used and the controversy therefore was known only by members of the military high command, the National Institutes of Health, and some of the researchers involved with the project.

Russia, an agricultural nation, may have experimented with so-called recreational drugs like cocaine, but we now know that the stimulant they chose was a safe one—ginseng. In fact, much of our present knowledge of ginseng comes from those Cold War experiments.

The Native Americans knew of "gisens" long before the European explorers arrived. They used it to treat bronchial disorders and neck and stomach pain. Today, we apply the technical name *Panax quinquefolius* to what is known as American ginseng.

In Asia, where ginseng had long been used to boost energy and overcome weakness (properties the Russians tested), ginseng has various names. *Panax ginseng* refers to the Chinese and Korean varieties, *Panax japonicus* to the Japanese, and *Eleutherococcus senticosus* to the Siberian plant. But no matter its origin, the uses and effects of the plant are the same.

The primary use for ginseng, especially *Panax* and the slightly less potent Siberian ginseng, is as an adrenal tonic. It is capable of enhancing performance, especially when the person is tired or is faced with complex tasks requiring careful attention. It stimulates the pituitary gland, causing it to release the hormone ACTH (adrenocorticotropic hormone), which combats stress, as do certain pharmaceuticals like prednisone, which are in the family known as corticosteroids.

Panax ginseng has also long had a reputation for improving sexual performance, which is one of the reasons people look for this form, usually sold as Chinese or Korean ginseng. The trouble is that there are no scientific studies on ginseng concerning the enhancement of sexual activity in humans. Some animal studies show an increase in testosterone and sperm levels, as well as more active mating behavior. Humans, however, are probably going according to faith, not fact. They also may be responding to the tonic nature. For most men, the safest and surest sexual benefits come from saw palmetto, which can be taken daily and is excellent for the prostate.

Ginseng is known as an adaptogenic substance. This means that it stabilizes some vital functions. For example, if you have high blood pressure, it lowers it to a healthy range. If you have unhealthy low blood pressure, it raises it to a safe level. This is all in addition to its benefits in increasing strength and endurance, and handling stress.

It is very important that you do not consider ginseng to be the equivalent of Kyolic garlic. Ginseng must be seen as a medicine to be consumed for short periods of time, not as a daily supplement. It is not like vitamin C, which you can take in quantity day after day. Instead, as the Russians discovered, it can be safely used for fifteen to twenty days, but then should be set aside for a couple of weeks before it is used again, if the need arises. You should never take high doses for a long period.

Note: Like pharmaceuticals, ginseng has side effects that you must keep in mind. The proper quantity to take will vary with your physiology and may differ from what is appropriate for a person of similar build and age. Among the possible side effects for everyone are anxiety, hypertension, insomnia, irritability, and nervousness. Women may also experience breast pain and changes in their menstrual pattern. These side effects should alert you to lower the dosage of ginseng you are taking or stop it entirely.

And ginseng is not for all conditions. If you are hypoglycemic, you should leave it alone, though small doses are probably safe. By contrast, diabetics often find ginseng extremely helpful. It lowers the level of the hormone cortisol in the bloodstream. Since cortisol interferes with insulin function, lowering its presence is of great help.

Ginseng is sold in a variety of forms. You can find it in an oil base and as granules for tea. You can obtain the whole root or root pieces, some of which are untreated and others of which are blanched. It is available as a liquid extract and as a concentrate. It is sold in tablets, capsules, and as a tincture. No matter how you buy it, make certain it comes without sugar or added color.

There are several factors about ginseng to be considered when choosing which form to purchase. If you've ever studied wine, you know that differences in the location of the vineyard, the type of soil, the exposure to sunlight, and the amount of rain affect the taste of the same type of grapes grown on two different plots of land. That's also true of ginseng. In what soil was it grown? Mature ginseng takes years to grow. How old is the root you bought? Which parts of the root were used? And what was the preparation? All these will determine its effectiveness, and in many instances they are not easy to determine.

When you read the label, look for a standard amount of the active ingredient. For example, the active ingredient of *Panax ginseng*, meant to help the adrenal glands, is ginsenoside. The recommended minimum for this purpose is 15 milligrams of ginsenoside a day, taken either in one dose or in up to three smaller doses. And always remember, if you can't find a knowledgeable professional to consult about ginseng, the watchword is caution.

GINKGO BILOBA

Ginkgo biloba and saw palmetto have probably done more to improve the lifestyles of elderly men than have all the pharmaceuticals combined. This is because saw palmetto can enhance their sex lives and *Ginkgo biloba* can make certain that they don't forget the pleasure they've had.

All right, I'm being playful. But with all the talk about Viagra and all the fear of Alzheimer's, it's nice to know that there are alternatives to what many people once assumed were the inevitable consequences of aging. And as numerous newspaper and magazine articles have touted of late, *Ginkgo biloba* helps you retain your memory. But to look on *Ginkgo biloba* so narrowly is to miss the true value of this natural remedy.

First, let's see how *Ginkgo biloba* aids your memory. The substance that comes from the ginkgo plant's leaves is rich in the terpenes (unsaturated hydrocarbons) known as bilobalides and ginkgolides. These nearly unpronounceable substances aid the flow of blood in the capillaries, the narrowest of the blood vessels.

Capillaries are so tiny, it does not take much to clog them. For many people there comes a time when the blood flow is not full enough to cleanse the capillaries of the toxins that flow through them. The poisons build up, especially in the brain. Even worse, the buildup of toxins means a buildup of free radicals, which damage the capillaries and the tissues normally fed by them.

The terpene substances in *Ginkgo biloba* help to open the passageways, flushing out the toxins and restoring circulation. This increases the oxygen and nutrient supply to the brain and the spinal cord, the components of the central nervous system.

The importance of this cannot be stressed enough. In addition, *Ginkgo biloba* removes toxins and free radicals from the network of blood vessels, nerves, and tissues in the eyes. Since, for many adults, aging means a gradual and needless loss of vision, the ginkgo extract is a boon. It may eliminate the degeneration of your eyes, maintaining or even improving your vision.

Have you ever had the frightening difficulty breathing caused by an asthma attack? You were experiencing the effects of free radicals on the alveoli—the tiny sacs in the lungs or on the lungs' capillaries that hold air. Free radicals can damage them to the point where an asthma attack is triggered. But *Ginkgo biloba* can counter all or most of these problems, preventing or lessening the effects of asthma.

Using *Ginkgo biloba* makes it easier for you to breathe, reduces the hardening of the arteries, enhances concentration, and even restores circulation to areas of the brain that have been damaged by a stroke. This is why it improves your memory and why it alleviates depression in many people, since the depression is often linked to problems of the circulatory system that the extract can counter.

Ginkgo is successful in treating other circulatory problems as well, among them chronic dizziness (vertigo) and ringing in the ears (tinnitus). Many migraine sufferers also find natural relief with this extract.

Ginkgo biloba is well understood as a natural medicine through both its use over the last five thousand years and through recent scientific studies. It comes from the oldest tree on the planet; records of its use date back to 2800 B.C.E. It is also one of the oddest, at least as we think of plants. Just as *Ginkgo biloba* helps humans sexually, so it has a sex life of its own. Some plants are male. Some plants are female. (Biloba means "two lobes," a description of the leaf's appearance.) Unless insects act as go-betweens, the plants do not reproduce.

What is less clear is the exact nature of ginkgo's effect on the brain. Some researchers dismiss much of its value because it is impossible to prove a direct effect, even though people who use it enjoy improved reasoning skills, memory, and ability to function.

The most recent information, facts I have confirmed in my practice and with colleagues who use natural remedies, is that three factors affect your brain as you age. First, and perhaps most surprising, the brain is more like a muscle in its needs than like a computer whose "hard drive crashes" after eighty or ninety years. Muscle strength comes with exercise and is lost with inactivity. There is a health spa cliché that you have to "use it or lose it," which means that if you don't exercise your muscles regularly, their strength and bulk will disappear. The brain is similar. New mapping procedures prove that the more mentally active you are, the better your brain will function. Deterioration is, in large measure, a consequence of inactivity.

You've undoubtedly seen a situation like this: Two people work together in a factory, office, or other location for forty or fifty years; each is looking forward to retirement. Both are in good health, and they have similar family histories. When they retire at the age of sixty-five or seventy, they both can look forward to at least one or two decades of life.

One man decides that he's worked long enough; retirement will mean a chance to relax. This person deliberately becomes sedentary, watching television programs, going fishing, maybe even spending time with children who live in different parts of the country. Overall, he has little activity that is mentally stimulating.

The second man sees retirement as an opportunity to try

something he's long wanted to do. If he does watch television, he does so for a short time and in an active fashion, that is, with one or two friends or family members. They gather to view a program, perhaps on public broadcasting or one of the cable channels featuring documentaries, and discuss what they're seeing. They find that the shows stimulate conversation instead of hushing it. This mentally alert man may enroll in an adult education program, a community college, or a university course; he'll take advantage of discussion groups, participate in social issues like the environmental movement, or volunteer to tutor in schools. He reads books, solves crossword puzzles, visits museums.

In recent years, as computers have become more sophisticated, people who enjoy keeping up with the latest technology are turning over their slightly older models to organizations around the country that put the computers in senior citizen centers, church meeting halls, nursing homes, and other places where the retired gather. (There is little resale value in outmoded machines.) The elderly are taught how to use electronic mail and keep in touch with younger family members and new friends more easily than by relying on regular mail or the telephone. Quite a few are going on the Internet and exploring chat rooms, where they can "talk" about their favorite topics, seek new opinions, and keep their minds busy.

What we discover when we compare the retirement of these two people is that the man who is active retains far sharper mental powers; that mental inactivity is actually destructive to the brain. Of course, this doesn't mean that you have to engage in brisk mental activity at all times. You can benefit from some sedentary time, because some quiet activities are important for the body. People who fish, who care for beloved grandchildren, who enjoy gardening or quilting may not be stimulating their minds while doing these things. They will, however, be relaxing their bodies, finding the peace that is essential for their well-being. It is the balance that is healthy.

Today so many people are involved in second careers, adult classes, and other mental stimulation that we can no longer correctly use the past definitions of aging. Studies have found that an eighty-five-year-old person in good health can handle all the tasks of living alone—shopping, cooking, paying the bills, cleaning—as well as someone of twenty-five. So now we talk about young old age (sixty-five to seventy or eighty) and old old age (over eighty or eighty-five). And even those standards are not always accurate, because much depends on the caregivers' ability to stimulate their charges in ways that prolong good health. Many nursing homes and extended-care facilities have been criticized when the presumptions of their youthful staff members do not match the potential of the residents.

What is important is that the brain be exercised. This is the first and most urgent factor in avoiding the symptoms that, through misdiagnosis, are often attributed to senescence, Alzheimer's, and other conditions.

The second vital concern is the circulation of blood in the brain. Unless rich, oxygenated blood moves through the capillaries, the mind will deteriorate. Someone with poor circulation will have difficulty thinking no matter how hard he tries to stimulate himself. And it is the *Ginkgo biloba* that stimulates this blood flow perhaps better than any natural remedy.

The third concern—not really within the scope of this book, but mentioned for completeness—is phosphatidyl serine, or PS. (Sometimes I think we scientists come up with such difficult terms in order to prove how smart we are!) PS is manufactured by the brain to maintain the health of the cell membranes. Unlike the hormone produced by the pineal gland, which eventually is no longer needed, large quantities of PS are necessary and normal throughout life. It is when the brain is unable to make enough of it that there's trouble, because the lack of PS is related to deficiencies of such essentials as vitamin B_{12}, folic acid, and the essential fatty acids.

People who experience deterioration of memory are often effectively treated with PS. Obviously they must continue to be mentally stimulated. And obviously, their circulatory systems must be healthy. In the past, however, many doctors using natural remedies have focused solely on the use of PS to the exclusion of *Ginkgo biloba.*

PS acts directly within the brain. It is in all brain cells, and the supplements, when needed, enter those cells. It regenerates nerve cells and cell membranes in ways that *Ginkgo biloba* cannot. But this is not an either/or matter. *Ginkgo biloba* contains terpenes and flavonoids, and acts as an antioxidant. Certain degenerative conditions of the mind associated with aging, therefore, can be slowed or stopped for prolonged periods with its use. Alzheimer's patients have routinely benefited from the use of ginkgo in double-blind scientific studies; their cognitive skills remained unchanged, but those of the patients on the placebo declined. And always, if the circulatory system is not strong, the brain cannot be healthy. *Ginkgo biloba* stands alone as a remedy and, for specific conditions, should be used in conjunction with PS.

Because our population is rapidly aging, Alzheimer's has become a disease as feared as cancer. The trouble is that Alzheimer's is difficult to diagnose and difficult to predict. It seems to start when a person is in his forties, though this is not at all certain. In many instances, it is misdiagnosed, sometimes because the person has been placed in a nursing home where inactivity, the absence of full-spectrum light, and a vitamin B–

deficient diet high in sugar are the order of the day. This person has the signs of permanent mental deterioration. It is true that mental degeneration from a variety of causes does afflict many people, but we have to remember that it can be prevented, postponed, or even reversed.

I believe that everyone should consider *Ginkgo biloba* a natural remedy in the preventive category. If you start to take it now, even if you are in your twenties or thirties, you will ward off severe oxidative brain damage. You will have a healthy blood flow to your brain. Your memory will be keen. You will be alert and relaxed. You will find old age a time of greater independence than you might have thought possible.

ALLERGIES AND *GINKGO BILOBA*

We learned of the importance of *Ginkgo biloba* when describing its effectiveness in preventing or reducing asthma attacks. Actually, ginkgo reduces the severity of most allergic reactions.

Our bodies contain a chemical we call a platelet activating factor (PAF). It is summoned into use whenever your body needs to spur the immune system into action. For example, if a germ attacks your body and an infection localizes the germ, PAF begins to work. The same is true when your nose runs or you're bleeding, waiting for the blood to clot.

A little PAF goes a long way. Allergic responses create abnormal situations. The bronchial tubes tighten when you have an allergic reaction to dust or other airborne particles. You secrete an excess of mucus, and get that miserable, drippy, disgusting feeling, all too familiar to those with allergies. Sometimes breathing becomes difficult. And all because of an excess of PAF.

Here's the key. *Ginkgo biloba* blocks the PAF, thereby lessening or eliminating the allergic reaction. Truly miraculous! Ask any allergy sufferer who has tried ginkgo. Why don't more doctors suggest ginkgo for patients with allergies? Because of the anecdotal nature of the treatment.

We do know that excess PAF creates a problem. Ginkgo apparently blocks the PAF. But people who are plagued by allergies don't always know when they're going to be exposed or, sometimes, when they've actually been exposed to particulate matter or whatever triggers their reactions. If they could predict the exposure, they could avoid it. All they know is that in the course of a year they may have a dozen or more (sometimes many more) allergic episodes. The way we judge the effectiveness of *Ginkgo biloba* for these people is by having them try it over the long term. They keep track of the frequency and severity of their attacks and then compare their experience with what they routinely suffered before taking the extract as a preventive. The anecdotal evidence has shown positive results of 100 percent, but the scientific evidence, based on examinations of the brain and the circulatory system, cannot deliver statistics for allergies.

SELECTING GINKGO

One way to get *Ginkgo biloba* into your system is to make a tea from the leaves. They're easy to obtain, and the tea is easy to make. It has only one drawback. *Ginkgo biloba stinks!* There's no nice way to put it. Just like skunks, the male and female ginkgo plants were made for each other, because no one else would want them. They have an odor that reminds me of rancid butter. If you make a tea from the leaves, you'd better have a terrible sense of smell.

By contrast, a standard ginkgo extract, available in health

food stores, drug stores, and some supermarkets, has no odor. If you shop around, you'll find that the price can be extremely low. I've found that between 80 and 150 milligrams a day suffices for most people and most problems. Look for 24 percent flavoglycoside content.

Chapter Six

CHELATION THERAPY

THE STORIES WE HEAR are often regional, not part of a national concern, so it is easy to overlook dangers that may pertain to all of us.

An Arizona family drives south into Mexico to purchase pottery. One brightly colored pitcher is so beautiful, the family uses it as part of their cookware. They wash it, fill it with orange juice, and delight in its appearance on the table each morning as they have breakfast.

Over time, members of the family notice changes in themselves. They have difficulty thinking. They have frequent, often severe headaches. Their behavior seems to others to be much like that of people with brain damage or brain defects.

The youngest children are apparently the sickest; their attention spans drop, their school grades slip, their movements are clumsy. By the time the children have been seen by a doctor, who does tests to rule out brain tumors and other problems, the children have suffered what may prove to be a permanent loss of intelligence.

Finally, and only through the process of elimination, the physician isolates the problem. The family is afflicted by lead poisoning, whose source is the brightly painted pitcher. The pottery was painted with a lead-based paint that, because of the citric acid in the orange juice, contaminated the juice. When the family members drank the juice, they ingested the lead and were poisoned.

Similar tragedies have occurred in the East and Midwest to families who bought older homes. The paints used in those houses were lead-based, and over the years, as chips of the paint accumulated on a windowsill or elsewhere, small children got them on their fingers and into their mouths. Sometimes the danger was spotted in routine screening procedures during regular checkups. When that happened, the situation was quickly rectified before long-term damage had been done. At other times, the damage was noted only after the child had become permanently brain-damaged.

Another source of metal poisoning is the older piping used in plumbing. The lead joint solder, the flecks of copper, and other trace metals, as we saw in the earlier chapters, are carried to the water we ingest through drinking and cooking.

Even in communities where trace metals are not so common, the environment can be a factor. Some business operations release particulate matter into the air, and we breathe it in. It is often invisible, tasteless, and odorless, or so familiar that we think the air is "normal."

Calcium can create another problem that we often overlook. You've been taught, probably since birth, about the value of calcium. "Drink your milk," your parents said. "It will give you strong bones and healthy teeth."

Women going through menopause are told to increase their intake of calcium, so they may chew antacid tablets loaded with calcium, or drink milk with every meal. They may conscientiously eat such calcium-rich foods as kale and broccoli. After all, they have been warned about the decline in bone mass that accompanies age. It is far better for the elderly, including men, to combine their increased calcium intake with weight-lifting exercises. Even light barbells are effective.

The problem is that calcium can also work against you. This isn't to say you shouldn't have it; of course you should. Calcium is the most abundant mineral in the body, where 99 percent of it is in the bones. But, like water, which can save your life or kill you through drowning, calcium has a negative side.

One of the most serious problems associated with calcium is its role in the formation of arterial plaque. This is composed of fats, cholesterol, and other substances that, when bound together by calcium, adhere to the walls of large and medium-sized arteries. The thicker the layer of plaque, the smaller the opening through which the blood can flow.

Many people wonder if they are susceptible to this problem. They assume that it is caused by other factors, especially fats. However, the truth is that anyone who is antioxidant deficient is potentially facing this problem. The antioxidants are what prevent the plaque from originally forming and growing. This means that you can follow a low-fat diet you are convinced is healthy, but if your antioxidant level is wrong, you will not be safe.

At first you may not notice any problem. Then, you may have pain or a feeling of tightness in your chest. The pain can radiate to your left side, afflicting your left arm, jaw, or chin. Maybe you become tired or short of breath. And if the problem is mild enough, you may decide that you've been working too hard. In fact, you are suffering angina pectoris or perhaps a full-blown heart attack.

Our understanding of aging has changed so radically, it is no longer unusual to see men and women in their fifties and sixties actively participating in a variety of sports—aerobic workouts in a health club, games of tennis and softball, jogging, or running. Business activity seems more intense these days, and more people work longer hours than at any time in the past. It's become normal in our culture to feel tired. Fatigue is almost a badge of honor, proof that you're working and playing hard. As a result, the symptoms of plaque buildup are ignored. You may have a heart problem that goes undiagnosed because its symptoms are attributed to your lifestyle.

In milder forms, the heart disease first seems to be heartburn or indigestion. So you swear off the ultra-hot salsa and chips. You forgo Cajun cooking. You eat in Chinese restaurants, ordering only the milder dishes. And all the while the plaque, glued together by the calcium, gets thicker and thicker, making your artery passages more and more narrow. Paradoxically, the calcium that is essential for good health has become a detriment.

Other circulatory disorders manifest themselves as we age, like gangrene of the extremities. So we always return to the need to rid the body of the excess minerals that have become the enemies of good health.

One way to get rid of excess toxins, metals, and minerals that work against our health is chelation therapy. This is a minimally invasive therapy; you do not have to undergo surgery, with all its risks. Instead, you can undertake oral chelation therapy, which means using a product that is sold over the counter, or you can have an intravenous administration of a chelator (EDTA), which must be done by a doctor, and which I'll soon explain.

For years, surgery has been advised for patients suffering

from the chest pain known as angina. A person with angina cannot be physically active without experiencing a painful squeezing or pressure in the chest. Arteriosclerosis, the blockage by plaque of the arteries carrying blood to the heart, means that the heart is not getting the necessary oxygen.

Angina is extremely dangerous and requires close observation by your doctor. The condition, traditionally, is treated by medication until such time as surgery is deemed necessary. Then the patient undergoes coronary artery bypass surgery or coronary artery dilation (angioplasty). Both procedures are frequently successful, but surgery is a trauma to be avoided if at all possible.

The danger inherent in the surgical treatment of angina, and of other heart problems, is that the chest must be opened while the patient is under anesthesia. Any surgery performed under general anesthetic is considered "major" and potentially life-threatening. No one is certain how the patient will react; patients have been known to die from the anesthetic. The risk is small—and surely less than what accompanies an avoidance of necessary surgery—but it is still a problem.

As you can imagine, "cracking the chest"—opening the chest to expose the heart—is traumatic for the entire body. It also exposes the patient to the risk of infection, both during the surgery and during the recovery phase, when drainage tubes are temporarily left inside the body.

Additionally, the heart-lung machine, a blood oxygenator and pump that is used whenever the heart is stopped for surgical procedures, creates problems for surgery patients. When the heart is to be started up again at the end of the surgery, it is shocked so that it begins beating, and the heart-lung machine is turned off. Unfortunately, the machine acts like a blender during the pump run, battering the red blood cells and, in a number of instances, doing long-term damage. It can also cause abnormal clotting of the blood that is being returned to the patient's body. Small emboli (blood clots) may form and make their way to the brain, causing minor strokes. Some patients, when they become conscious again, find that their memory of loved ones, work skills, and other critical knowledge has been impaired. Many regain the knowledge. Some require therapy. And some are those whose families are grateful that the patients are alive, yet are deeply saddened by the extreme changes in their loved ones' personalities.

These days, much of the heart-lung machine damage has been obviated by the use of anticoagulants both before and after the operation. The anticoagulants minimize the clotting problems but may cause other difficulties because of their blood-thinning properties, if they are not taken in precise doses. And that danger is present if the patient is confused, as is sometimes true of the elderly and those who have had minor strokes.

Finally, anyone who has heart surgery is likely to experience depression for up to two weeks after the procedure. This is a biological response. The recovering patient may begin to cry for no reason, sometimes in the midst of an activity that should not make her sad at all. This is not serious, but, again, it is something we'd all like to avoid.

These are some of the reasons that an operation should be avoided if there is a safe and reasonable alternative.

Chelation therapy, or ethylene diamine tetraacetic acid (EDTA) therapy, the technical name for the slightly invasive procedure, handles some angina problems with little risk. It is based on the knowledge that there are certain chemical substances that act as chelators. They latch on to the foreign substance and remove it from the body.

EDTA is a chemical given intravenously that acts as a chelator. There are other substances you can take by mouth, such as garlic, vitamin C, and pectin, that act as chelators. The intravenous chelation method is far more effective.

Do you remember when the different kinds of superglue were introduced? Some of the ads showed a car suspended in the air while attached to a crane by a single drop of that great glue. When you went to the store for the product, you were reminded that the risk of someone gluing himself to a table or chair was so great that you'd better also buy a container of a chemical that would neutralize the glue. It was actually a kind of the acetone used as nail-polish remover, and it could weaken the glue's bonding strength.

In arteriosclerosis, calcium is the strong glue holding together the cholesterol, fats, and other substances that form the artery-clogging plaque. Chelators act like acetone, in the sense that they bind with the calcium and help flush it from the body. No calcium, no biological glue. The plaque breaks up and is safely flushed from the body, and your arteries are unclogged without surgery.

The reason that EDTA chelation therapy may be unfamiliar is that cardiologists are not routinely taught it. Instead, they are taught to recommend invasive cardiac procedures. One of the first challenges to the idea that invasive procedures must be used to treat angina came from Dr. Thomas Graboys, writing in the November 11, 1992, *Journal of the American Medical Association.* Dr. Graboys, a Harvard cardiologist, studied 168 patients with angina who had been told they needed an angiogram, an arterial catheterization procedure used to visualize the heart and its blood vessels. This is an invasive procedure.

Dr. Graboys first worked to confirm the diagnosis by echocardiogram (sound waves), an exercise stress test, and by having each patient wear a heart monitor for twenty-four hours. When he was done with all 168 patients, he found that 134 did not need the catheterization. With the others, who had more severe problems but were not faced with an immediate crisis, he tried such methods as changing their medication for the next two months. At the end of that time, only six patients proved to need the angioplasty.

Dr. Graboys's point was that invasive techniques are often not needed. Although he was not advocating EDTA chelation, that method might well have worked for most of the patients studied. The other six simply had hearts that were so badly damaged there was no alternative.

This is most important! It is now known that patients whose hearts are still healthy may experience complete blockage of the coronary blood vessels, and they can do extremely well without surgery.

EDTA chelation therapy not only helps to flush out the plaque-forming calcium deposits from the blood vessels, it also gets rid of excess copper and iron. And this is important, because, as we saw, copper and iron are minerals that, in excess, encourage the formation of free radicals, which may endanger your arteries. So EDTA performs two vital functions in one procedure.

In fact, oral chelation therapy for the treatment of circulatory problems caused by toxic metal accumulation is considered safe and valuable. It is being used to treat Alzheimer's disease, arthritis, multiple sclerosis, and Parkinson's disease, and it is proving extremely effective, according to both doctors and patients. Although much of this rests on anecdotal evidence, even the most vocal critics cannot specify any problems.

Intravenous EDTA chelation therapy is a different matter. There has been some controversy surrounding this treatment, of which you need to be aware. First, a bit of background. When a treatment is developed by a pharmaceutical company, a patent is issued for a limited period of time. As long as the company holds the patent, it is in its financial interest to find as many different ways as possible for the treatment to be applied. The EDTA patent was originally held by Abbott Laboratories, which aggressively pursued its uses until the expiration of the patent, approximately thirty years ago. Then, with EDTA in public domain, the company had no incentive to continue its research, so it turned its attention to other areas, leaving EDTA to the private sector. Unfortunately, the private sector's research grants frequently come from pharmaceutical companies eager to support work on the patented products, not the ones that would bring them no profit. As a result, no large sums of money were made available to study EDTA. In addition, EDTA chelation therapy did not win the support of cardiovascular surgeons. If you make your living by cutting, you're hardly likely to promote noninvasive procedures.

The one counter to the decline of both experimental and practical study of EDTA chelation therapy came in 1972. At that time, a group of physicians who used EDTA chelation therapy formed the American College for the Advancement of Medicine. Their purpose was to educate others. This is one of the reasons that the therapy has survived and is beginning to gain more recognition.

In all fairness it must be mentioned that there was a period when EDTA therapy caused kidney failure leading to death.

The chelator was injected too rapidly, and a toxic factor in it damaged the kidneys. But this was in the early stages of research and use.

With time, the proper procedure for EDTA chelation therapy was specifically described, and for more than a decade the Food and Drug Administration has backed studies on its safety. From what I have read, there have been more than a half million instances of EDTA chelation therapies, without a single fatality, and most of them without any adverse side effects. Also, there is solid evidence that it is an excellent treatment for many types of vascular disease as well as cardiac angina. Most of the criticism I have seen does not take into account the extensive research findings on the safety and effectiveness of EDTA chelation therapy over the past several years.

EDTA chelation therapy, it must be said, is not to be started on a whim. First, you must undergo a thorough physical examination, including tests for kidney function, cholesterol, blood, liver function, electrolytes, and glucose. You should have a chest X ray and an electrocardiogram; you should have your mineral and vitamin B_{12} status analyzed. Some of the studies, including those on kidney function and blood, will usually be repeated throughout the chelation therapy.

How EDTA chelation therapy is administered will vary with your condition. Typically, you will have two treatments a week, each of three hours' duration. And you will be given nutritional supplements, depending on your needs. They usually include trace minerals, vitamin C, and magnesium. Probably during the course of the therapy you should be fortifying your body with B-complex vitamins, zinc, and chromium, in addition to whatever other vitamins and nutritional supplements you're currently using.

• • •

For any problems requiring chelation therapy, you can begin to help yourself by changing your diet and your approach to nutritional supplements. During the chelation therapy itself you will add the essential minerals that are being displaced. You should have iron from a natural source, like blackstrap molasses; you should have alfalfa, kelp, and zinc supplements. The zinc supplements, please note, should be accompanied by sulfur-rich foods, as zinc inhibits the action of sulfur. You can counter this with legumes, onions, and garlic, all rich in sulfur.

Your basic diet should be of the type recommended for people with heart disease or high cholesterol. You'll want to add fiber-rich foods and distilled water, as well as a high-protein drink or a supplement containing the essential amino acids. Be certain your supplements are complete ones. Amino acids, for example, are fully effective only when the supplement contains them all. They do not work well alone.

Your diet should also be rich in manganese, because it is a chelating agent that blocks calcium from entering the cells of the arterial lining. Whole wheat, buckwheat, dried split peas, Brazil nuts, barley, and pecans are all good sources of manganese.

Finally, if you have trouble getting information on chelation therapies, you'll find a good source of referral in the American College for the Advancement of Medicine, P.O. Box 3427, Laguna Hills, CA 92654.

Chapter Seven

NATURAL
HORMONE MAINTENANCE

THE TRUTH ABOUT WOMEN and medicine is that, for the past few centuries, research has viewed women as second-class citizens. Men were the doctors. Men were the researchers. Men were usually the test subjects, and most doctors assumed that all bodies functioned like the "ideal" one—theirs.

Not that the researchers were fools. They did know the difference between male and female anatomy. They understood the existence of a complex chemistry that allowed a woman to become pregnant, carry a baby to term, give birth, and supply all essential nutrition for the first few months of the baby's life. Yet the standards for diagnosis and treatment were largely based on male physiology, and, as a result, many women needlessly suffered physical problems or died because of the ignorance of the doctors.

Oddly, this was not the case historically. During the time of Luke, the physician and writer responsible for two of the books of the New Testament, his medical contemporaries were mostly women. The first century A.D. saw the application of extensive medical knowledge among the Romans, and most of the doctors of that time are believed to have been female. In fact, so advanced was what they knew that almost every surgical procedure carried out by American doctors in 1950, including eye surgery, had been done in first-century Rome. The difference, and it was a critical one, was that the ancients had no knowledge of antiseptic practices. They could perform excellent technical work in many instances, but their patients died from infection. And this problem haunted physicians and surgeons until the middle of the nineteenth century, when Joseph Lister discovered the concept of antisepsis.

The aging of women, through hormonal changes, is considered shameful by many in contemporary American society. Women are embarrassed by the onset of menopause, and women of "that certain age" are sometimes viewed as discards. This is why the heroines in films are rarely over forty, though men a decade or more their senior are considered romantic leads, despite sagging, bagging jowls and gray hair. This is why older women in business are considered volatile leaders when they assert themselves, but younger women, who make the same astute comments are derided as "comers." This is why there is an industry prepared to cut and sew, suck fat, inject collagen, and generally turn a woman's skin into a stiff, taut parody of nature, all in the name of fighting aging.

When women returned to the medical profession early in this century, they were not able, at first, to change the way research was handled. They were encouraged to go into family practice or to be pediatricians, obstetricians, or gynecologists. They were not directed to do research, nor were they welcome in such aggressive and "macho" fields as surgery. As a result, they helped their women patients as best they could, relying on what worked for themselves. But they made little change in medical treatment.

In the 1950s, when medical research was breaking new

ground, women were still perceived as second-class citizens, even though these same women had enjoyed a brand-new freedom and lifestyle during World War II. In those years, due to the shortage of civilian men, many women left the countryside, journeyed to the big cities, got jobs in shipyards and steel mills, manufacturing plants and construction businesses. They drove trucks, carried mail, and often filled high-paying jobs previously denied them. But when the war ended and the men returned, there was an effort on the part of many established citizens to re-create the past in a world that was no longer the same.

In the 1950s, the spread of superhighways and the sudden appearance of flourishing middle-class suburbs resulted in a new culture. Women were no longer considered for responsible jobs; they were relegated to lower-paying ones. Most people now lived in cities and suburbs, not the rural areas of their youth. And the work ethic saw men leaving home early to commute to their jobs and returning late. The suburban ethos had the wife acting as mother, cook, cleaning woman, chauffeur, and a myriad of other roles. She would usually feed the children before their father came home and then prepare dinner just for him.

In a sense, suburbia became a collection of single-parent homes. The mother was with the children all week. On weekends, the father was expected to see to chores around the house, go to church, and rest. His involvement with his children was secondary.

A look at the popular culture of the 1950s will show why, when medical research took off (allegedly there were as many medical developments between 1950 and 1965 as there were from the start of recorded medical history until 1950), women were not included. They were considered addle-headed and unpredictable. The title character in *I Love Lucy*, created by Lucille Ball, was only a slight exaggeration of the perception men had of their wives, daughters, and sweethearts. Cartoons, television shows, and movies all played with this idea. Stimulants, tranquilizers, and sleeping pills were disproportionately prescribed for women, and magazines devoted space to the volatility of females, especially when they reached menopause.

Birth control had less to do with women's choices and reproductive rights than with men's freedom to have sex whenever they chose to. Sexually transmitted diseases were rampant, but few thought of condoms and birth control pills, which became available in 1961, as being related to health. Rather, condoms and similar "protection" for young men were meant solely to prevent babies. The men tried to "score" without an "accident."

This relegation of women to second-class status meant that medicine was slow to deal with breast cancer, ovarian cancer, heart disease, and other disorders in women. Drug experiments were frequently performed on men, and their effect on women was largely ignored, which is why the "harmless" thalidomide caused thousands of women to give birth to deformed infants despite the drug's having undergone extensive testing.

The birth control pill brought new problems. Never before in history had women utilized hormones in the manner they could with "the Pill." While it changed society, ushering in the sexual revolution, where casual sex among several partners replaced the previous generation's belief in sexual monogamy, it also endangered many women. Those who suffered from migraine headaches had more severe episodes. Sometimes when that happened, the failure to stop the Pill resulted in a stroke.

Diethylstilbestrol (DES) was another wonder drug of the postwar years. From 1945 through 1971, women who were likely to miscarry and those with gestational diabetes (diabetes whose onset occurred during the pregnancy) were given DES with wonderful results. Women who had lost one or more children to miscarriage brought their next babies to full term. Women who had experienced the unpleasantness of the diabetic reaction remained healthy. Even better, science found that DES made a wonderful fattener for animals. And since the drug was used to feed livestock, almost every man, woman, and child in the nation was getting the drug.

Why was the drug not used after 1971? Enough time had passed for science to learn that DES, actually a synthetic estrogen, caused numerous problems. Women were having reproductive disorders and a tendency toward immune disorders. Men had a reduced semen and sperm output, as well as development problems of their reproductive organs.

Today we have improved contraceptive pills and implants. Women are conversant with estrogen, progesterone (progestin is the name of a synthetic), and testosterone from the time they're in their teens. Many are taught to look on their bodies as a chemistry set that came without a few vials of critical substances needed to work the formulas. Instead of the woman's body being viewed as a natural manufacturing plant that can be stimulated through appropriate diet, pharmaceutical companies encourage women to believe their bodies are unnatural and somehow inferior to men's. It is as though God made Adam, and then subcontracted the construction of Eve to General Motors on a day when the plant workers went on strike after lunch. Everything she needs is built in, but nothing works quite right and everything must constantly be fine-tuned.

The result is that many doctors and pharmaceutical companies make large sums of money by fueling fears and neurotic behavior among women. Among the myths propagated are that menstruation is shameful, ovulation is abnormal, and the monthly changes in biochemistry are somehow threatening. (The latest edition I've seen of a psychiatrists' handbook lists premenstrual stress as a mental illness.) And menopause is a life sentence that hangs over every woman. In fact, women can't cope with their lives without the external chemistry provided by pharmaceutical companies and delivered by doctors. It's as though no women lived full lives when doctors weren't around to inject them with hormones. It's as though good health is not possible for the female. And perhaps the greatest tragedy is that many women listen to this nonsense: The issue of hormones is rarely explained or understood.

The same is increasingly true for men, as is exemplified by the recent craze for Viagra. Consider the following: When a man is a teenager, he can have several orgasms a day, and there are periods of a youth's early puberty when he is thinking about sex an average of once a minute, according to researchers. Erections are frequent. Nocturnal emissions are common. And masturbation may be a fairly common means of relieving sexual tension when he's alone. As with women, body chemistry changes with age, and sexual satisfaction increases. The older male is much better able to sustain an erection and please a woman, who comes to her greatest feelings of sexuality later in life. Foreplay lengthens. Ejaculation before the woman reaches orgasm is less likely to happen. And his emotional pleasure is more intense than he had imagined in youth. Yet the fear of not being able to perform as frequently and well as he would like has led many a man to grasp at Viagra and testosterone injections even though he has a normal, healthy sex drive. The results for some men have been adverse reactions, including fatalities.

Yet we know that men who have minor problems with sexual function can overcome them in a number of nonpharmaceutical ways. First, since the testicles need to be cool to function best, switching from briefs to boxer shorts is all that some men need. Others seek a cooling-down period following such exercises as bicycle riding, which warm the testicles. And still others find nutritional alternatives such as saw palmetto, vitamin E, zinc, and the like, combined with a moderate change in diet and exercise, are safe ways to enhance erotic ability.

The difference between men and women is that men only recently have been targeted by pharmaceutical companies. Thus, it is only now that they have become so worried about what is a natural part of their lives that they look for ways to change it.

HORMONAL IMBALANCE

The first time most women are aware of hormones in a noticeable way is the onset of menstruation. Most women will have some form of premenstrual symptoms a week or two before the start of menstruation—cramps, anxiety, nervousness, backache, breast swelling, usually accompanied by tenderness, headaches, insomnia, water retention, abdominal bloating, food cravings, depression, fainting spells, acne, skin eruptions, and personality changes. These last range from outbursts of anger to drastic mood swings, thoughts of suicide, and, in the extreme, violent behavior.

Mood swings are the most serious for many women and the greatest cause for jokes and bias. In fact, for many years women were excluded from positions of responsibility because PMS would make their functioning "impossible" under pressure or in a crisis. A woman could not become President of the United

States, we were told, because PMS would limit her ability to deal with rapidly changing world conditions. "Would you want someone in a blind rage because her period is approaching to have her hand on the nuclear trigger?" was asked of those who suggested female candidates.

The latest statistics we can find show that approximately 5 percent of all women have PMS symptoms severe enough to be incapacitating. We have also found that 30 to 40 percent have symptoms severe enough to interfere with their day-to-day lives. Yet all of these problems can be reduced or eliminated, mostly through changes in diet and exercise.

The hormonal imbalance that is the usual cause of PMS is an inadequate amount of progesterone and an excess amount of estrogen. This often brings about the retention of fluids, which may seem a minor problem until you understand that the retention adversely affects circulation. Oxygen cannot readily reach the brain, the uterus, and the ovaries.

Diet is a factor in hormonal imbalance and the consequent reaction. Meat and dairy products can contribute to the imbalance, because so many animals are fed hormones to speed growth or stimulate milk production. The problem is exacerbated when women worried about the diminution of bone density increase their consumption of milk.

Note: We are talking about meat and dairy products, not calcium sources in general like broccoli and kale. Hypoglycemia, malabsorption, food allergies, and other problems are also associated with PMS. Vitamin and mineral deficiencies, clinical depression, and erratic levels of beta-endorphins are further problems.

The beta-endorphin issue has only recently come under study. The term may not be familiar to you, but if you exercise heavily or have ever heard an athlete talking about "hitting the wall," you know what beta-endorphins are. These narcotic-like substances are produced by the body to lessen pain and discomfort.

Long-distance runners encounter beta-endorphins when they hit the wall, meaning they've reached the point where they no longer feel discomfort. At first many runners experience only the stress of running. They are conscious of each stride, they're breathing hard, and they often have a burning sensation in their lungs. As their muscles ache, they're probably asking themselves why they decided to enter the race or do the present workout. Suddenly, they feel good. They're still breathing hard, but they no longer have the desire to quit. They feel as though they could maintain the pace all day if they have to. They've hit the wall.

What has really happened is that their bodies have begun to produce the natural painkillers beta-endorphins, the same natural drug produced during childbirth to ease labor pains, the same natural drug produced during sex, when the friction of intercourse might be uncomfortable for the woman without it.

My recommendation for women with PMS symptoms who want to counter them with natural remedies is to eat plenty of fresh fruits and vegetables, whole grain cereals, beans, breads, peas, nuts, seeds, lentils, broiled turkey, and fish. High-protein snacks should be eaten between meals.

Drink at least a quart of distilled water daily, starting a week before the menstrual period and continuing through a week after. This is in addition to your normal liquid consumption.

Do not eat salt, processed foods, "junk" or fast foods, and red meats. If you don't want to abandon them entirely, refrain from eating them one week before the expected onset of symptoms. Remember that salt will contribute to that bloated feeling and water retention.

Eat fewer dairy products. They block the absorption of magnesium and increase urinary excretion. Refined sugar also increases magnesium loss.

Avoid caffeine, which is linked to breast tenderness. It is a diuretic and can increase anxiety.

Ideally, do not consume alcohol or sugar in any form during the week before symptoms are expected. These cause you to lose valuable electrolytes such as magnesium through excretion.

You might also consider a fast of fresh juices and spirulina for several days before the anticipated onset of menstruation.

The concerns about estrogen and progesterone are again experienced at menopause. Doctors, pharmaceutical companies, and feminine-care product advertisers usually focus on estrogen, because the natural estrogen decline can affect a woman's physical appearance, always an easy target in our culture.

During the years when the matter of birth control introduces you to estrogen, it's easy to assume that the hormone is related solely to reproduction. Estrogen receptors, however, are found not only in the vagina and bladder, but also in the skin, bones, brain, breasts, arteries, heart, and liver. This is why some women going through menopause find that their skin is no longer taut. It becomes coarse and may sag as its moisture content, stimulated by estrogen, diminishes.

Far more serious is that postmenopausal women develop the same risk of heart attack that men have developed a decade or so earlier. Estrogen reduction may be a contributing factor.

The reason is that the ovaries are the source for most of the body's estrogen before menopause. But during menopause—

which may last as long as five years—the ovaries' output sharply diminishes. The ovaries still work, but the other organs known as the endocrine glands now supply most of the estrogen you'll use the rest of your life.

The most important thing to remember is that menopause is not a disease; it is a natural change that can be physically exhilarating if you address the change through diet and supplements. It is not the end of youth and sexuality, though it does mark the end of your childbearing years. In fact, some women report a healthier sex life because they now have the freedom to enjoy it without the risk of pregnancy. Many men are delighted to find that their wives become more sexually aggressive following menopause, as the psychological concern of pregnancy is gone and the joys of adult sex in a committed relationship can be experienced as often as desired. The fact that a lubricant such as coconut butter oil might have to be used because of vaginal dryness resulting from estrogen reduction is considered a minor concern. It is also known that for some women, increased sexual activity ends the vaginal dryness problems.

Having gone over all of this, let's look at the different hormones with which you are or will be concerned. Let's also discuss the sometimes controversial topic of natural hormone-replacement therapy.

HORMONES

The simplest definition is that hormones are chemical substances produced by the endocrine glands. The pituitary gland at the base of the brain, so small that it's about the size of a pea, produces nine different hormones. It also acts as a coordinator for other glands, monitoring the hormone levels in the blood and making the appropriate adjustments.

Then there is the hypothalamus, located directly under the brain, near the pituitary gland; the thyroid gland, in front of the "Adam's apple" in the neck; and the parathyroid glands, the adrenal glands, the pineal gland, the testes or ovaries, the thymus, and the islets of Langerhans in the pancreas, all of which produce hormones. Together, they form the complex chemical system that regulates many functions of the body.

In a healthy system, all the parts function well together. If there is an excess of hormones, however, the rate of cell division can be altered in harmful ways, often leading to cancer of the breast, uterus, or other organs. And this is why tampering with the natural cycles of a woman's life can actually endanger her health. Yet we do have evidence that hormone-replacement therapy, carried out appropriately, can be beneficial. We'll begin by looking at some of the concerns related to the fluctuation and regulation of the hormones in a woman's body.

CANCER RISK

Remember when I mentioned how little research has been done on the unique biochemistry of a woman's physiology? There is much we now know, but much we don't understand.

For example, your risk of getting breast cancer is, in part, directly related to your onset of menstruation and of menopause. The earlier you menstruate and the later you reach menopause, the greater your risk of getting breast cancer, because you receive a high dose of estrogen throughout this period.

What does this mean for you? Possibly nothing. For many years American women began to menstruate around the age of eleven and reached menopause around the age of fifty. Breast cancer rates were relatively predictable, and when they were higher than average, the reason was often a genetic predisposition in the women of that family.

Today all this is changing. For reasons related to estrogens released into the environment (another problem of our modern society), girls are starting their menstrual cycle as young as eight years of age. Not large numbers yet, but there's no question that girls are beginning to menstruate much earlier than in the past.

Menopause so far remains stable, occurring when a woman is around fifty years old. If, however, that changes, and women continue to produce estrogen until a later age, then the breast cancer risk will go higher.

We have also learned that pregnancy is a factor in breast cancer. Society cannot tolerate teen pregnancies. No matter when a girl has had her first period of menstruation, if she becomes pregnant before she is eighteen, she will be greatly protected from breast cancer. A woman who delivers her first baby after she is thirty-five is three times more likely than a twenty-five-year-old to develop the disease. Also, women who have several pregnancies are more protected against breast cancer than women who have few. A woman who never becomes pregnant has the highest risk of all, other factors being equal.

This is not to say that I think all women should get pregnant during their teens and then have lots of full-term babies in order to avoid breast cancer. Such a situation may be ideal for your hormones, but it is not realistic for our society, our culture, or the planet. We live in a time when you are likely to have no children or a family of two or three at the most. You are likely to have educational and work goals and commitments that keep you from getting pregnant until you're in your thirties. You may feel you should limit or abstain from childbirth in order not to tax our planet's resources. And you are likely to have started menstruation earlier than your mother and grandmother did.

Many changes that affect your hormones during pregnancy are outside the scope of this chapter. Now I want to discuss those situations that most women encounter, as well as those that pertain to hormone reduction at menopause.

ORAL CONTRACEPTIVES

Depending on your age, the time of your first sexual relations, the age when you started menstruating, and your doctor's suggestions, oral contraceptives have been a part of your life for many years or are a subject you are now considering. The following information is related to the hormone content of such birth-control methods. If you've been taking the Pill for a while, or if you're thinking of starting it, you should understand the risks.

First, no one can say with certainty that oral contraceptives cause problems, although much of the available information shows that there is a slightly increased risk of breast cancer among women who take them, and that risk is greater for young women in their late teens who rely on high-progesterone contraceptives. After five years the women have a four times greater chance of getting breast cancer than women who are over twenty-five when they start the Pill. For all women, there is a risk of several forms of cancer if their contraception involves injections of medroxyprogesterone.

The dangers reported, however, do vary with the studies. And a few studies show a reduction of the risk of endometrial and ovarian cancer in women who take the Pill. There may be a higher risk of heart attack and cardiovascular illnesses, though the data are still sparse.

It is important to understand that our knowledge of the problems presented by long-term use of oral contraceptives is relatively new. In addition, we are faced with the problems created by the increased life expectancy of women today. In 1900, women were not expected to reach sixty years of age. Women in their mid-fifties were considered old; most women barely passed through menopause before dying.

A hundred years later, women routinely live into their mid-eighties. Problems building slowly in the body that would not have been revealed in the year 1900 are major causes for concern in the year 2000. We are now presented with a broader horizon, and have to take into account the long-term effect of our choices. We are also trying to avoid creating new problems through hormone therapies for menopausal women that may diminish the quality of old age.

HORMONE-REPLACEMENT THERAPY

The efficacy of and need for estrogen and other hormone-replacement therapy is argued among medical professionals. For some, the therapy is simply another example of women being treated as if menopause were a disease. The natural is being declared unnatural. Normal physiological changes are being viewed as symptoms of illness.

And the truth is that many women experience no problems with menopause. They are comfortable and happy. They may even find it psychologically liberating, an attitude reflected in their behavior toward both their spouses and their jobs.

Those women who do have problems usually fit one of two categories. The first are those who have been educated to believe that menopause is a time that requires regular medical attention, in the same way a pregnancy does. They schedule regular appointments with their physicians, regardless of symptomology, and start use of one or more medications.

The second are those women who are less concerned with the physical sensations or consequences of menopause but are alarmed by the depression they feel at its onset. They feel "over the hill." Such women often undergo what might be called menopause harassment, jokes about the aging process, about the lessening of their desirability, and about the dull quality of their life. "Turning fifty, are you?" is a typical comment. "Guess your husband will be turning you in for two twenty-five-year-olds." Unfortunately, our society has brainwashed many women into believing that it's one short stop from menopause to senility, walkers, nursing homes, and all the handicaps of age.

We see, too, that the aging of the baby boomers has done much to break these stereotypes. These days many women over fifty find themselves in demand because of their wisdom, life skills, and freedom from the responsibilities of rearing young children. Many of them are experiencing a second marriage, where they feel sensual and sexy, and many are discovering that they still attract the physical interest of men older, younger, and the same age.

But before this awareness began to take hold in America's consciousness, the myths of male and naïve youth dominated popular culture. Advertisements warned women facing menopause to lay in a supply of denture cream, support bras, facial creams, and other poultices, potions, and magic spells. They were given the subtle, insidious message that they had to do whatever was necessary to hide their years. These shattering experiences led many to experience a depression their doctor termed menopause-related. Because the condition required medication, their sadness was reinforced. It was these conditions that gave rise to hormone-replacement therapy.

That is not to deny that there are women who need hormonal rebalancing. Many have had glandular problems most of their lives. Many are seeking short- or long-term hormone relief from an unusually difficult menopause. And many see only the positive value of estrogen-replacement therapy, and never look into its possibly negative side effects.

This is why a better understanding of natural hormone therapy can save your life. What you know when you go to your doctor will help you to monitor your care, suggest alternatives, and alert you if there is reason to seek another opinion.

ESTROGEN

Perhaps the most publicized reason for you to seek estrogen-replacement therapy is your wish to decrease the risk of osteoporosis and cardiovascular ailments. What is less known is the full meaning of estrogen, its relationship with progesterone, and how their interaction affects various aspects of your health.

First, let me dispel one of the biggest myths of estrogen replacement: that estrogen supplementation will reverse osteoporosis. When your hormones decline, your bones may become thinner and more brittle, greatly increasing the possibility of your incurring injuries to your hip and spine. By taking estrogen, you will slow or stop the deterioration of the bone mass. That does not mean that you can reverse the process and rebuild your bones.

Osteoporosis can also be prevented or slowed by your doing regular exercises, especially with weights, and consuming adequate quantities of calcium. Adding estrogen will heighten the effects of these measures, but estrogen without exercise and diet changes—ideally, before menopause and continued throughout the rest of your life—will have little effect.

Note: Other hormones do have an impact on bone regeneration after menopause. Among them are progesterone, testosterone, and DHEA, which I'll define later.

Another prevalent myth is that all the problems of menopause are caused by hormone loss. Frequently, there are physical changes that we mistake for hormone-related problems, as with vaginal irritation and dryness (atrophic vaginitis), a condition that can be alleviated by estrogen replacement but is not necessarily caused by estrogen loss. But it is more important that you avoid substances that dry the mucous membranes, which means that you should give up caffeine and alcohol. It may also mean that you should not take antihistamines and diuretics as often as you may have done in the past.

Soy foods added to the diet may help not only atrophic vaginitis but hot flashes as well, and may aid in preventing a higher risk of breast cancer. This is why, when considering the safest way to deal with changes in body chemistry, lifestyle adjustments may be more important than hormone replacement. These changes and supplements will be discussed in greater depth later in this chapter, but for now let's take a look at the makeup of estrogen and the role it plays within a woman's body.

The word "estrogen" actually refers to a group of related hormones, of which estriol, estrone, and estradiol are the primary components. At different phases of your menstrual cycle, the amounts of each component will vary. Estriol makes up between 60 and 80 percent of estrogen at any given time. Estradiol and estrone make up 10 to 20 percent of estrogen, fluctuating within these normal ratios.

Progesterone is the hormone that works in balance with estrogen by countering much of its most worrisome side effect, the possibility of increasing your risk of cancer. We now know that the greatest danger of estrogen-replacement therapy is the failure to balance it with a proper amount of progesterone. Your taking one without the other increases the risk of cancer in much the way that a teenager's taking the progesterone-rich birth-control pill raises her risk of cancer in later life.

A popular form of prescribed estrogen, Premarin, consists primarily of estrone rather than estriol, and has a lower amount of estradiol (and sometimes tiny quantities of other hormones) than is found in human estrogen. It also has some equilin, a hormone extracted from the urine of pregnant mares.

Yes, horses. The fact is that the meaning of "natural hormones" varies with the manufacturer of the product. I think of natural hormones as being the replacement of a woman's own hormones. But pharmaceutical companies argue that a female horse is "natural." So truth in labeling is not challenged. What you need to consider is whether you are comfortable taking a "natural" estrogen if that product is not originally from and for humans.

Note: If you are concerned with medical ethics and animal rights, you may be interested in learning that the method of obtaining equine estrogen used to make the prescription product for humans is uncomfortable for the mares. They are put in special stalls that allow for only limited movement during the time when their urine is rich in estrogen. Sometimes they can't lie down, and sometimes they're given less water than they should have so that the urine will be thicker and richer. If you've never thought about the source of estrogen you're taking, this information about the mares may be a reason to avoid animal-based sources. Of course, this is a personal choice, but one you can make only if you have all the facts.

Missing from the popular replacement is estriol, which was eliminated for the same reason humans make many medical blunders. Researchers sometimes forget that there is a logic to all creation. If God gave it to us, there is a reason, and our not knowing what that reason may be does not lessen something's importance.

For years researchers thought estriol was not particularly important, so they concocted the estrogen replacement without it. What they neglected to do was look at the long-term effect of this change.

Remember when I said that progesterone may counter the cancer-causing property of estrogen? We now know that estriol plays a major role in this. If you take a natural hormone replacement that does not contain estriol, you may increase your risk of cancer. Nature balanced human hormones to keep you safe. The moment we diverge from the exact duplication of a human hormone, we may be adding unacceptable risk factors.

In recent years, estrogen patches to be worn on the skin have become popular. So far, they seem to be safer than oral estrogen replacements, and they usually contain the estriol, estrone, and estradiol combination instead of the substituted equilin.

ANDROGENS

Most people think of a hormone as being either a male property or a female one. By this reasoning, estrogen is for women and the androgens, like testosterone, are for men. In fact, estrogen and androgens are found in men and women. The adrenal glands produce both hormones, and a woman's ovaries produce not only estrogen but also testosterone. The difference, of course, is the amount of each hormone in each sex.

Androgens are an issue in hormone-replacement therapy because of their importance to a woman in her daily activities. Testosterone relieves many of the symptoms of menopause, like vaginal dryness and hot flashes, for which we normally think of using estrogens. By counteracting vaginal dryness, a woman's sexual pleasure is enhanced.

Earlier, I referred to the hormone DHEA without explaining what it does. DHEA, or dehydroepiandrosterone, is a precursor to the androgens. It peaks at the end of adolescence or early adulthood, usually at age twenty-five to thirty. From then on it diminishes so rapidly that someone fifty years old has only a fractional amount.

DHEA has two functions, which is why it is now considered a part of hormone-replacement therapy. Some of it is metabolized into estrogen and testosterone. The rest acts as an antioxidant, and hence a preventive of cancer and heart disease, and it is now thought to be involved in preventing the buildup of fat. It performs the latter function because it aids in creating muscle mass. It also stimulates bone growth and is a factor in fighting osteoporosis. The fact that when you are eighty, you probably have in your body only 10 percent of the DHEA that you had at twenty-five indicates that many of the problems of brittle bones associated with aging may be directly related to the lack of DHEA.

Most of the studies of DHEA I've seen concerned men. The DHEA effects include significant reductions in the risk of heart attack, body fat reduction without weight reduction (maybe not ideal for those of you who judge your health by your weight, but important for your health), and the reduced incidence of

Alzheimer's disease, multiple sclerosis, and stress-related illnesses. DHEA also seems to strengthen the immune system, improve memory, and possibly prolong life.

The hormone is available in both prescription and nonprescription forms. Disgenin is DHEA in a weak strength, made from wild yams. Other extracts from unprocessed wild yams are converted by the body into DHEA.

You may assume that stronger quantities are better, but new findings indicate that caution is in order. Some physicians now think that high doses of DHEA may have the serious side effect of reducing the body's ability to synthesize the hormone. In other words, the body seems to shut down when it is overwhelmed, so the prescription quantities cut down on what you actually get because they stop the body's natural production. In addition, animal studies show that high doses of DHEA may damage the liver.

DHEA-replacement therapy should be considered for premenopausal symptoms (ages thirty to forty). It should be conducted with care. It should also be handled only with the addition of such antioxidants as vitamin C, vitamin E, and selenium to avoid the risk of liver damage.

WHAT'S RIGHT FOR YOU?

Hormone-replacement therapy is obviously not a simple decision. First, consider your own body. What are your concerns, based on your body's changes, your family history, and other factors? What problems should you consider normal and transitory, if a bit uncomfortable? Remember that in the past two decades at least, many middle-aged women developed a dependency on medications because of the uncaring, time-pressured, or naïve physicians who treated them when they were teens. At that time, instead of discussing premenstrual changes, cramping, and the like, doctors routinely responded to complaints by recommending tranquilizers and minor painkillers. In a major scandal, ultimately addressed in Congress and a number of books, it was found that most of the teens needed nothing. The changes were normal; they just didn't understand what was happening to their bodies. Discomfort became to them a symptom of something severe. They felt they had to take the drugs, and soon they became psychologically dependent. Yet five or ten minutes of frank discussion between patient and physician would have resulted in the teenagers' living the same way that half the world's population lives, accepting the normal changes of the childbearing years. You must not let menopause or postmenopause be a period when a physician's time allotment per patient prevents you from gaining all the information you should have to avoid the problems once so common among teenagers.

You must explore your options with a physician whom you trust. You must recognize that synthetic hormones are often not effective, and that "natural" hormones must be studied so that you can tell what they actually are and thereby avoid something like the equilin-estriol trade-off. And you must remember that menstruation, menopause, and all the other experiences of being a woman are natural. This is the way God made you. This is the reason you have, on average, more stamina than the man. This is the reason you're likely to live longer than a man. This is the reason some cultures revered women and is also the reason that some cultures feared them and tried to make them feel inferior.

If you do decide to pursue hormone-replacement therapy, learn all the possible risks. Each medicine is packaged with an information sheet you should read. If it's missing, get this information from your pharmacist. In addition, insist that your doctor and your pharmacist go over possible problems with you.

Suppose, for example, that you're given a prescription for Estratab or Premarin, two of the more common brands of the natural estrogen made with equine estrogen. The information available to your doctor will show that it is an effective form of replacement estrogen for menopausal women. But it will also show that the potency is so great that it may cause metabolic changes in the liver. Worse, it probably should not be used by women who smoke cigarettes, are obese, have high blood pressure, varicose veins, and high cholesterol.

By contrast, most truly natural (not derived from horses) estrogens are completely safe and easily metabolized. These include estropipate and estradiol. Under the best of circumstances, though, estrogen alone is not a good idea. If you do take it, use the smallest possible oral dose, and, even then, take it only every other day.

There are two common ways to obtain the estrogen—orally and with a patch. The most frequently used patch is called Estraderm made by Ciba-Geigy. It is applied to the skin of the abdomen or the thigh. Some women have found it irritative and the patch had to be left in one place no more than three or four days before moving it slightly. It was also a nuisance when showering or swimming because it had a tendency to come off. However, when it stayed in place, it was convenient and allowed for consistent assimilation of the estrogens.

When you take the estrogen orally, it has to go through the liver. This may prevent a consistent assimilation. Both approaches obviously have their benefits and drawbacks, though the best form will allow consistent assimilation.

Progesterone is probably more important than estrogen. And natural progesterone is available as a cream, made from wild yams and available at most health food stores, which not only relieves menopausal symptoms, but also helps stimulate your body's natural regulation and production of other hormones, including estrogen. Just be sure to tell your doctor (though this is a form of self-medication about which I've heard of no ill side effects).

For many women, changes in diet and lifestyle will smooth the transition to menopause in a natural way. First, it's important to recognize that some of the problems of menopause can be prevented by the very activity some women and men may think should diminish. Vaginal dryness can, as we saw, be avoided by a greater frequency of sexual intercourse. If you're in a committed relationship, try to make time for frequent physical intimacy. Do not make it a pressured relationship, as is sometimes formed by young couples trying to have a baby. Rather, use it as a time of relaxed renewing of physical sensation, prolonging foreplay, enjoying each other's touch, and letting the sex act ease you through one minor side problem of menopause.

Raise the level of your natural painkillers, your endorphins, through regular exercise of at least thirty minutes a day, perhaps a brisk walk at lunchtime or before or after work. Or you may try a workout in a gym or health club. The important point is to do the exercise daily and for a period of time that will make certain the endorphins are working for you. The minimum weekly total of 3.5 hours has sometimes been found to eliminate hot flashes with no other treatment. In one study, women who were seriously considering estrogen-replacement therapy because of the severity of their hot flashes cured the problem with exercise. Equally important, exercise is critical in steadying bone mass and preventing or diminishing osteoporosis.

Phytoestrogens are substances that are rich in estrogen and will not cause some of the problems related to hormone replacements. (The prefix "phyto" indicates that the substance comes from plants.) Soy foods are among the richest in phytoestrogens, a discovery made during studies of Asian cultures, whose women consume at least two thirds of a cup of soy products each day and clearly experience estrogen benefits. Among the soy products sold in the United States are miso, tempeh, and tofu. Many large supermarkets and most health food stores stock soy hot dogs, soy sausage, soy cheese, and soy desserts, along with soy milk. Every so often a company will devise a recipe that calls for soy and is meant for vegetarians: The soy version of chicken croquettes is an example.

Other phytoestrogen foods are celery, nuts, seeds, parsley, and fennel. The last one is extremely rich in compounds that act like estrogen.

You can also reduce vaginal dryness and irritation by avoiding alcohol, antihistamines, caffeine, and diuretics. The elimination of such products from your diet and the addition of both phytoestrogen foods and exercise may well grant you an easy passage through menopause.

The American Indians discovered that the herb black cohosh was excellent for curing menstrual cramps and for eliminating hot flashes, depression, and vaginal atrophy during menopause. They passed their knowledge of the herb to women colonists, who relied on it. Later, scientific studies of black cohosh confirmed what the Indians had known. The herb cuts down what are known as luteinizing hormone levels, giving it a strong estrogen effect. Eventually, the knowledge became international, and women in Germany who seek a natural alternative to estrogen therapy are prescribed Remifemin, the registered trademark of a black cohosh formulation. It is available in the United States as Remifemin too, but you can also obtain it as a powdered root or a tea. Generally it should be taken two or three times a day to be most effective.

Asparagus contains steroidal glycosides, which help in the stimulation of hormone production and have been found to counter the anemia caused by folic acid deficiency.

AFTERWORD

Hormone maintenance is fundamental to ensuring a long and healthy life. Although hormone-replacement therapy can be extremely beneficial, doing nothing more than making sure that your diet, exercise regimen, and supplementation are appropriate can be the perfect answer. Only you can decide on the best program for you, based on the information contained here and on discussions with a doctor you trust.

The essential point is that none of the natural passages through human existence should ever be considered a disease, an abnormality, or a medical problem. Hormonal changes are part of life. They are not illnesses to be cursed, feared, or conquered through pharmaceuticals. All phases of life are good. Enjoy them.

Chapter Eight

VITAMINS
C AND E

IF THE MANUFACTURERS of prescription drugs have suffered one disappointment during the last fifty years, it's that they didn't invent vitamins C and E. The more we learn about how these potent antioxidants benefit our bodies, both independently and together, the more we appreciate their value. If you're playing America's favorite game of Russian roulette—smoking cigarettes—you may be able to delay the damage to your body by taking C and E, and in that way buy enough extra days of life to come to your senses and give up smoking. Then keep up the vitamins, because they'll help restore your lungs to a level of health you haven't experienced in years.

Recovering alcoholics, who need the B-complex vitamins in order to detox effectively, also find vitamins C and E essential for rebuilding the cell walls of the liver and blood vessels. In fact, the deaths of some of the most famous alcoholics in the entertainment industry, like Peter Lawford, the brother-in-law of President Kennedy and a member of the Frank Sinatra–led Rat Pack, were caused primarily by a vitamin C deficiency. His once athletic body had been severely damaged from years of abuse, and he had become jaundiced from his liver problems, but it was likely the lack of vitamin C that caused him to bleed to death through the walls of his blood vessels. They could no longer contain the blood, a condition often seen by pathologists.

Vitamin C prevents scurvy. Recent studies suggest that vitamin C, along with zinc and large quantities of water, shortens the common cold to as little as two days. Vitamins C and E, working together, affect your sex drive, your eyesight, and numerous other functions. Yes, just imagine if they could be controlled by the manufacturers of prescription drugs . . .

In truth, an attempt was made to have the Food and Drug Administration (FDA) declare vitamin E a pharmaceutical. That was in the late 1970s, and the manufacturers' goal was to prove vitamin E a possible danger and have it removed from health food stores. How could they do this? Since vitamin E is fat soluble, the drug manufacturers hinted that a casual user might overdose. What they didn't mention was that there were no such cases that they could cite. The companies' real concern was that vitamin E was doing such an excellent job at improving the cardiovascular health of men and women, reducing the risk of cataracts, and providing so many other benefits, that there was a risk of their products being prescribed less often. Too many people were healthy!

The idea was as ridiculous as that of the cigarette manufacturers' attempt to convince the American public that cigarettes weren't addictive, didn't cause cancer, and that all the negative claims were as yet unproven. This, after almost a century of evidence to the contrary.

Our understanding of vitamin C predates our understanding of vitamin E, because we knew of the problems that its absence caused in sailors on long voyages. Its history is both old and new. Back in 1747, the British Navy was plagued with scurvy. The sailors were weak, anemic, bleeding from their mucous membranes, and unable to perform their duties. A Scottish physician named James Lind was assigned the task of correcting the problem, which he deduced was caused by a lack of citrus fruits.

Dr. Lind's theory was valid, and the crews that followed his advice were fine. But it wasn't until 1800 that the British Admiralty accepted his recommendation. At that time, citric acid in the form of lime juice and lemon juice, which could be readily stored for the long voyages, became part of the daily diet of sailors. By 1806, there were only two cases of scurvy in the British Royal Navy. A quarter century earlier, before the doctor's discovery was heeded, there had been 1,457 cases.

In the Pacific Northwest, explorers were so horrified by the natives' custom of sharing thin slices of moose testicle that they refused to partake. What they didn't realize was that these people were trying to save their lives: No other source of vitamin C was available in the frozen land. We don't know how the natives discovered that their health was dependent on this vitamin C–rich portion of the moose, but they did. Their willingness to share it with outsiders was important, yet many an early settler grew sick and died, because he found the source too unpleasant. Only years later, when vitamin C had been isolated, did we understand that the ritual sharing was prized for its life-saving value.

Understanding the role of citrus fruit and other sources of vitamin C, including the moose, wasn't the same as isolating the chemical factor. That discovery was made by Albert Szent-Györgyi, who isolated ascorbic acid in 1928, and was awarded the Nobel Prize for medicine in 1937.

In the 1960s, Dr. Jonas Salk, widely heralded for his discovery of the polio vaccine, began discussing the merits of vitamin

C in fighting the common cold. Today we understand that it is also a powerful antioxidant and helps protect us from environmental pollution.

The antioxidant property of vitamin C is vital to us. Pollutants in the air and water regularly produce the free radicals we talked about earlier. Vitamin C not only neutralizes many of the free radicals to which we are unavoidably exposed, but helps combat voluntary free radical damage—cigarette smoking.

As deadly and dangerous as cigarette smoking can be, vitamin C can ease smokers through their folly. Smokers who raise their intake of vitamin C reduce the damage done to the immune system more than do smokers who don't use supplements. The latter have huge drops in their serum vitamin C levels, a depleted store of antioxidants, and a higher susceptibility to cardiovascular disease, cancer, and other sicknesses. This is not justification for smoking while taking vitamin C; the results are deadly either way. Vitamin C just slows the problem. It is, however, a reason for those exposed to secondhand smoke, like restaurant workers, to boost their vitamin C intake.

Perhaps the oddest story of an overwhelming need for vitamin C supplements occurred in Northern California. Richard Chase, a serial killer eventually known as the Vampire of Sacramento, blamed his murderous rage on the failure of vitamin C to cure his problem. He believed that his mother had fed him laundry detergent, which turned his heart to stone. (He did not understand why hospital emergency room workers dared claim they could help him when all they did was send him to the psychiatric ward. He was not crazy! They were delusional.) His solution was to cure his condition with vitamin C.

Chase, knowing that there were different forms of the vitamin, decided that the best was in the freshest fruit he could get. So every morning he bought fresh oranges, wrapped them in a scarf, and wore them on the top of his head. In this way, he was certain, he would obtain all the benefits of the vitamin. No one knows whether Chase continued to believe this, because he accidentally killed himself when he overdosed on the antipsychotic medication he had been hiding away after he was sent to jail for his murders.

The Nobel Prize winner Linus Pauling popularized the consumption of megadoses of vitamin C when he stated his belief that the vitamin was the ultimate wonder pill: It would keep you healthy, prevent or cure the common cold, and in general fight every ailment. He used to keep his pockets filled with vitamin C tablets, and take one every time he was interviewed. His proven genius, his enthusiasm, and his evangelical fervor stimulated new research into all phases of the vitamin.

Pauling may not have been wholly accurate in thinking vitamin C the peerless panacea, but the experiments he inspired did prove that this simple vitamin is of major importance to your health. And it can ease high-stress experiences like chemotherapy for cancer, making them less dreaded.

Although your body needs vitamin C, it doesn't produce it. Fortunately, there are numerous supplements, some better than others. Only chewable vitamin C should be avoided because, effective as it is for your body, it's not good for your teeth. Plain vitamin C is not as good as estified C (ester-C), which links ascorbic acid with dietary minerals like potassium and calcium and is absorbed more readily in the body.

The megadoses recommended by Linus Pauling were as high as twelve to fourteen grams a day, but there's a risk, at that level, of kidney stones and other difficulties. The time when such a high dose is warranted is during the extreme stress one encounters when undergoing chemotherapy. Most people, fortunately, never reach a level of intake that would cause problems, because vitamin C is soluble in water. The worst that could happen is that we'd have enriched urine. I personally take 2000 milligrams of ester-C every day.

Vitamin E has a less colorful history than vitamin C, in part because so many foods contain it that a person would be hard put to acquire a deficiency! It wasn't people, it was laboratory rats, a traditional source of new medical information, that led researchers to isolate vitamin E. In 1922, a study showed that rats fed a diet without vitamin E were unable to reproduce. Only after wheat germ oil, rich in vitamin E, was added to their diet could they once again bring forth more rats.

Problems with sexual activity may be eased by vitamin E. In 1978, Bernard Green, Ph.D., a Manhattan therapist who later wrote extensively about nutritional alternatives to stimulants and depressants, closely watched the progress of a patient who underwent a prefrontal lobotomy in a mental hospital. The man was well enough to function in society, but he found he could no longer be sexually active. He had a girlfriend, but he couldn't ask her to marry him, because he'd lost the ability to have an erection.

Dr. Green had already altered the man's lifestyle by having him adopt a healthier diet, take long walks, and learn about certain basic nutritional supplements. When he heard of the new problem, he had the patient double his vitamin E intake to 1600 IU a day. Within a week, the man's sexual function was restored. He maintained the higher dose for a reasonable period, then cut back to 1200 IU a day. And he never again reported a problem with intimacy.

Just because vitamin E is found in more foods than vitamin C doesn't mean you should neglect supplements, although it would be easy to draw this conclusion because the effects of too little vitamin E manifest themselves only over a prolonged period. What adds to the confusion is that when signs of a deficiency begin to show, they are more likely to be looked on as symptoms of some mysterious illness rather than as a lack of vitamin E. That's why we have no dramatic stories of navies and explorers, madmen and major research breakthroughs, as we do for vitamin C.

What Richard Chase didn't know was that if it was his heart that was in trouble, vitamin E should have been his preferred cure. The higher the level of E in your blood, the less likely it is that you'll die of heart disease.

Vitamin E is in fact not a single vitamin, as vitamin C is. It's a combination of eight chemicals divided into tocopherols and tocotrienols. Of the two groups, the more important is d-alpha tocopherol, a funny term when you learn that its Greek origin means "bearing children."

Vitamin E is soluble in fat ("lipid soluble," in technical language) which means that it lingers in fatty molecules and cell membranes. This is a highly beneficial quality, because it serves as protection against excess oxygen-forming free radicals.

Note: When you buy vitamin E, look for the natural source d-alpha tocopherol. You may find a synthetic form usually listed as dl-alpha-tocopherol, but the difference between the d and the dl is more than a single letter. Synthetic vitamin E is only half as effective as natural vitamin E at best, in large measure because the synthetic form is composed of eight chemicals, known as isomers, only one of which is the molecular equivalent of natural vitamin E.

The reason this chapter links vitamin E and vitamin C is that recent studies have found that the combination enhances the antioxidant effect of each. The following information on the use of vitamins C and E may make them seem like nature's wonder drugs. What is more remarkable than the ways in which these natural remedies work for you, however, is that we know so little about them. We're just beginning to understand the many ways in which they affect our health, slow the aging process, and guard us against many environmental dangers.

THE EFFECTS OF THE VITAMIN C–VITAMIN E PARTNERSHIP

Earlier, we discussed oxidation, the process by which a life-giving substance—oxygen—becomes an aggressor against your cells. Among the targets of oxidation are the mitochondria, or energy generators of the cell.

To understand what mitochondria do, think of your body as an energy plant. The basic fuel for humans is food used in the way that mechanical generators process coal, wood, nuclear products, or some other fuel, to produce energy. Next comes the digestive process, by which the food—fuel—is turned into smaller components for easier handling. These small components are metabolized; that is, broken down into still smaller elements. What started out as a steak or chicken, salad or vegetarian dish on your dinner plate is ultimately changed into material for the cells of the body to use.

In this final stage, the tiny structures the mitochondria, located in every cell in your body, produce the organic compound adenosine triphosphate (ATP), which is part of this process of creating energy in all living cells. The mitochondria are the structures that make it; they are the power plants of the human cell.

The trouble is that the older we get, the less efficient the mitochondria become. The brain, heart, and kidneys begin to slow down in their functions. Cells that earlier were able to repair themselves are no longer up to the task. Soon we notice the results in our physical appearance. The endocrine system produces lower levels of hormones, our skin becomes dry, our metabolism slows, we gain weight, store fat, and lose muscle tone.

It is important that you understand that there are a number of ways to counteract this. Twenty to thirty minutes of brisk cardiovascular exercise shortly before you eat will speed up your metabolism. Exercising with weights will improve your muscle tone. And changing your diet to reduce sugar, unnecessary fats, and junk foods will also delay the aging change. But change does and will occur. You can, at best, control only the timing and severity, which is something that wasn't known in the past, when older people were encouraged to slow down, relax, and enjoy retirement through sedentary living.

The slowing of the mitochondrial function, a significant part of the aging process, is affected by a reduction in your body's ability to counter oxidation damage. This is where vitamins C and E, often accompanied by beta-carotene and selenium, become critical. Otherwise, we all face a high risk of age-related problems, ranging from Alzheimer's to adult-onset diabetes to obesity and heart disease.

Vitamins C and E affect areas ranging from the important—diabetes and Alzheimer's—to the self-indulgent. In 1997, the *Journal of the American Medical Association* published an article on the relation between vitamins C and E and one's ability to enjoy the kind of meal that causes obsessively health-conscious people to cringe.

All of us know that high-fat diets are not good for us, and we also know that when we choose to indulge, we get tired. There have probably been days when you've walked to lunch at a fast-food restaurant because the fresh air, the sunshine, and the escape from the office made you feel good. Then you or-

dered something as self-indulgent as, say, a cheeseburger a
fries, savoring tastes you usually, and quite properly, deny
yourself. But even as you did this, you knew that you'd have to
eat "right" over the next few days to atone for your dietary
"sin." So when you walked back to the office, you probably
kept up a brisk pace and maybe added a couple of extra blocks
in order to "walk it off." Chances are that you felt great when
you returned to your office. What with the walk and the pleasure of forbidden food, you felt refreshed. But suddenly, within
minutes of sitting down at your desk, you began to feel sleepy.
If you could have gotten away with it, you'd have taken a nap.
But that was probably impossible, and you couldn't hide your
tiredness. For the next couple of hours your productivity went
down. And you may have taken frequent breaks just to keep
from falling asleep.

The problem passed within two to four hours, and you may
then have felt productive once again, so you ended up thinking
that maybe you needed more sleep. Or you thought that the
walk had tired you. And if you're like most people, you certainly didn't think that sleepy feeling had to do with the heavy
lunch.

The fact is, though, that blood flow slows down for two to
four hours after you've eaten a high-fat meal, and when that
happens, your body slows down, too. Sleep is a natural way of
getting through this period, which is why you felt tired. And
that's why some people, when they can, take a midday nap. But
none of this had to happen.

If you take vitamins E and C, according to the *JAMA* study,
your blood vessels will remain open, and the tired feeling will
seldom overwhelm you. Your blood flows normally, and an
occasional overindulgence will not pose as many problems.

Earlier we talked about plaque, made from oxidized fats,

.e walls of the blood vessels and narrows them. ᴶᵘᵉ hardens the vessel walls, further diminishing ᴵᵈ once plaque has formed, pieces of it can break ᴵ along the bloodstream, where they may block the sᴵᵁ ᴶels of the brain, heart, lungs, and other organs. Vitamin E, ᴬnd to a lesser degree vitamin C, combat this by "desludging" the blood, strengthening the lining of the arteries, and helping prevent lipid peroxidation. And not only can vitamin E inhibit the oxidation of LDL cholesterol in your blood vessels, but it appears to limit and possibly reverse the creation of plaque lesions.

Over all, vitamin E, taken in adequate quantities, has been shown to reduce deaths from heart disease. (This means 800 to 1200 IU daily, or slightly higher, which translates to two to three 400 IU capsules, the most commonly available form of d-alpha tocopherol.)

There is an amino acid, commonly found in the body, called alpha lipoic acid. This is a substance that enhances the effectiveness of vitamins C and E, both potentiating and conserving them. Because of its unique characteristic of being both water and fat soluble, it can go anywhere in the body. I have found that adding a tablet supplement of at least 50 milligrams but no more than 250 milligrams will greatly improve the effect of vitamins C and E. Within this range there are no known side effects, and I personally choose to take the highest dose in conjunction with 2000 milligrams of C and 800 IU of E each day.

CATARACTS

The older you get, the more you'll be hearing about cataracts. Ophthalmologists and optometrists will check for them each time you have your eyes tested. Friends will talk about their surgery or that of their parents. It is one of those problems of aging that everyone has or knows someone who has. At any given time, approximately four million people in the United States experience this degenerative disease, which can be stopped in its early stages. In fact, cataract removal is the most frequent major surgical procedure done each year for people receiving Medicare.

What exactly are cataracts and how do they form? The lens of the eye is normally clear; we can compare it to the sulfur-rich liquid of a freshly cracked egg, known as albumen (or egg white), which is, as you know, a clear liquid until it is heated.

Proteins in the lens of the eye, like the liquid of the egg, contain sulfur. Damage to these proteins, most often through too much exposure to the sun's ultraviolet light rays, causes them to become cloudy. This is no different from the egg's albumen, which turns white when exposed to heat.

Many people experience tiny cataracts that their doctors carefully monitor. They don't hurt our ability to see. They don't prevent us from reading or driving a car. The doctors simply watch to see whether they get worse.

Eventually some cataracts grow so large they can cloud the lens. At that point, one's ability to see is diminished or lost completely. To complete the egg analogy, it's like taking a fried egg, holding it up to the light, and trying to see through the white.

Traditional cataract treatment does not involve an aggressive effort to stop the degeneration. You may be told to wear sunglasses that block UVA and UVB light rays, but that would be about all. The doctors know that the clouding can move so slowly that a person may have cataracts for twenty years or more and never need an operation. If, though, the cataract does impair vision, surgery is the usual treatment.

Cataract surgery is most often done on one eye at a time in case something goes wrong. The lens is removed, and an implant is inserted in its place. But this is not the end of the problem. Cataract surgery may have to be repeated in a few years, and, what is more worrisome, the surgery can be a factor in a much more serious condition, macular degeneration. This involves oxidative damage to DNA, the degeneration of the capillaries, and the formation of scar tissue. These conditions cannot be reversed through natural remedies. All we can do is avoid or delay macular degeneration through the use of antioxidants. The risk of raising the chances of this disorder by cataract surgery shows how critical it is to avoid cataracts if possible.

Cataracts are caused not only by sunlight but by other free radical damage. The reason they are of particular concern to the aging is that when the pineal gland begins shutting down, reducing the available melatonin, free radical damage increases. If you smoke, have diabetes, or are exposed to radiation (including sunlight), the problem is exacerbated.

Cataract and other degenerative problems of the eye, along with some side effects of cancer therapies, have recently been thought to be alleviated by the smoking of marijuana. People who are not involved with the drug culture have lobbied their legislators to make the use of marijuana legal for medical purposes. But what they usually ignore is that smoking anything is injurious to your health.

It is fine to discuss the relative merits of alcohol and marijuana as recreational drugs, but neither is particularly healthy. And when scientists analyzed why marijuana genuinely helped some people, they found that it wasn't the marijuana; rather, it was an increase in the patients' melatonin output that had the beneficial effect. Equally important, even this benefit, brought about by the marijuana, was wasted, because the smokers used their "joints" any time of the day, and the melatonin benefit came at night when the pineal gland normally operates. You can safely boost your melatonin through supplements combined with vitamins C and E that will reduce your cataract problem.

The lens of your eye has a fatty outer lining, which can be damaged by lipid peroxidation. What is involved is hydrogen peroxide, a chemical whose effect can be minimized by the anti-oxidant glutathione. Glutathione comprises three amino acids—cysteine, glutamic acid, and glycine. Technically, it is known as a tripeptide, and it neutralizes the hydrogen peroxide in lipids. Although it's naturally produced in your body, its quantity, like that of melatonin, decreases with age. At the start of a cataract problem, there is always a seriously low level of glutathione in the blood.

Without glutathione, the hydrogen peroxide prevents the DNA of your eyes' lens cells from replicating. In a healthy eye, the new cells will be identical with the old ones. But after damage by hydrogen peroxide, the new cells are larger than the old ones and are irregular. They lose the ability to reproduce, and as the years pass, the lens become opaque and misshapen.

As I write this, it is not possible to reverse existing cataract damage. Instead, we look to long-term protection, and this is where vitamins C and E serve their preventive function.

In October 1977, the *American Journal of Nutrition* reported on the first full study of vitamin C and cataracts. The taking of vitamin C alone—but remember that I think you must take it in conjunction with vitamin E—drastically lessened the incidence of early cataracts. It was also a major factor in limiting the severity of the cases that either existed before, or arose during, the study. Of great importance was the study's finding that the short-term use of vitamin C is not adequate. The daily use of vitamins C and E supplements is a lifetime concern.

ly we believe that vitamin E helps to prevent cata-
e same way that it protects all of the body's fatty
ecause it is fat soluble, the vitamin penetrates the cell
and n.. eus wall, as well as the lens lining. And as it becomes
oxidized, it frees vitamin C to act as the lens' rejuvenator.

What does all this mean? The May 1998 issue of *Ophthal-mology* revealed that a good multiple-vitamin supplement can reduce the incidence of cataracts by a third. This is without medicine or surgery. Add vitamin E, and the reduction is by half. Add vitamin C, and the vitamin E becomes even more effective.

Note: There is a bioflavonoid that I find provides antioxidant protection against cataract formation: Quercetin enhances the absorption of vitamin C. Quercetin, found in blue-green algae, is available on its own as a supplement.

Remember that cataracts take years to develop. That is why the natural remedy should be considered for the long term: Fortunately, it helps many parts of the body. Just be sure to supplement the vitamins C and E with alpha lipoic acid and the bioflavonoids.

DIABETES

Vitamins C and E are not the most critical nutrients when treating diabetes, because the deficiency most often found among diabetics is that of chromium. In fact, it is the underlying concern of Americans who have any sort of blood sugar problems, from hypoglycemia, which affects two out of three people, to diabetes, which is a problem for an estimated fifteen million Americans, only a third of whom are aware that they have the condition.

Those with wide fluctuations in their blood sugar levels

may find chromium picolinate the preferred supplement. The exact dosage varies from person to person, though I find that between 200 and 400 micrograms a day work best. Its use must be monitored carefully by your physician, however, as chromium in supplement form will affect your insulin. For some people, it may have side effects, which vary with the brand of the supplement. The side effects range from a skin rash to light-headedness, either of which is an indication that you should stop taking the supplement until you can discuss the matter with your physician.

Fortunately, chromium is in many foods. Among them are brown rice, cheese, meat, brewer's yeast, whole grains, dried beans, blackstrap molasses, calf's liver, chicken, eggs, dairy products, mushrooms, corn oil, and potatoes. This means that most people can obtain what they need through an appropriate diet.

Before learning the fundamental ways in which vitamins C and E can help in treating diabetes, you have to understand the nature of the disease. There are three forms of diabetes. The first, diabetes insipidus, is the one with which you may be familiar if you were a child watching television in the 1950s. That was when diabetes was beginning to be understood, and various medical organizations were so anxious for the public to know about the problem that they ran informational advertisements on early television. These ads stressed the warning signs—extreme thirst, unrelated to physical activities, coupled with a high urine output, regardless of how much you may have been drinking.

Today we still talk about those warning signs, but we know they are related primarily to diabetes insipidus, not to diabetes mellitus types I and II, which were discovered fairly recently. We also know that diabetes insipidus is the rarest of the three forms of diabetes, caused by a deficiency of the pituitary hormone vasopressin or by the kidneys' inability to react appropriately to that hormone. This inability is usually the result of damage to the pituitary gland.

Of the more common forms, diabetes mellitus Type I has been called juvenile-onset diabetes, because of its frequent occurrence in children and young adults. The patient is insulin dependent, because the beta cells of the pancreas, the organ that manufactures insulin, have been damaged or destroyed, perhaps because of a virus or an autoimmune problem. Either way, the external source of insulin is necessary.

Some of the symptoms of diabetes mellitus Type I are similar to those of diabetes insipidus. Parents may find that a child is wetting his bed, usually a number of years after bed-wetting has stopped. He has abnormal thirst and frequent urination, and he may be losing weight, even though he's eating as much or more than ever. He experiences fatigue and nausea, sometimes accompanied by vomiting. These are all warning signs and symptoms that should not be ignored.

Type II diabetes mellitus often appears in adults whose family history shows the disease. In these cases, the insulin produced by the pancreas is ineffective in controlling the blood sugar, leading to fatigue, abnormal drowsiness, unusual thirst, blurred vision, skin infections, tingling or numbness in the feet, itching, and frequent urination (which, in a man, may lead to inflammation of the penile glans and foreskin).

Unlike diabetes insipidus, unfortunately, few of the symptoms are so unusual that the person seeks medical treatment. Some people may be diabetic for months or years, but they attribute their malaise to overwork, the pressures of a change in lifestyle—marriage, divorce, having children, relocating—or a lack of sleep. Only after a long period of misery do they suspect a problem and go to a physician, who diagnoses the condition.

Poor diet, we saw, is a factor in Type II diabetes mellitus. This often means too many processed foods, low in both fiber and complex carbohydrates. It does not necessarily mean a high-sugar diet, though eating large amounts of candy, cookies, pies, and cakes of course will contribute to the onset. Alcoholics and drug addicts are also susceptible, because so often they ignore a proper diet at the very time that their addiction places their bodies under high stress. Sugar is often an ingredient in many of their self-destructive indulgences, from alcoholic beverages to cigarettes. Because cigarette tobacco is sugar-cured, the craving for sweets that smokers have when they try to quit is often a sign of cigarette-induced hypoglycemia.

One side effect of this form of diabetes is the patient's inability to taste sweetness as readily as a healthy person. The diabetic tends to use far more sugar and other sweeteners because she cannot tell when she's had enough. In the drug addict going through detox, this form of diabetes may be overlooked for months unless his blood or urine is checked for diabetes.

You can begin to understand how essential vitamin C is for a healthy immune system when you understand that insulin helps to move it into cells. The diabetic with a shortage of insulin is likely to have cells deficient in vitamin C. That's why vitamin C supplements are critical for all diabetics. I recommend daily doses of between 2000 and 5000 milligrams of vitamin C with bioflavonoids.

When diabetes remains undiagnosed, or when the physician is unaware of the need to increase the vitamin C in the diabetic, other problems show up. Cuts and scrapes have a tendency to bleed abnormally and heal slowly. Vascular disease may be evident, with ischemia (poor blood flow) and gangrene. Cholesterol levels frequently rise, and the immune system is depressed. And there may be glycosylation of proteins and the accumulation of sorbitol, factors that lead to eye and nerve disorders. As little as 2 grams of vitamin C a day added to your supplements can reduce or eliminate these problems.

Vitamin E also prevents many of the complications of long-term diabetics and it improves insulin action. Since vitamin C helps boost the effect of vitamin E, the combination of the two seems to reduce oxidative stress. Perhaps more important for those who don't have the disease but may have a tendency toward it, the vitamin E supplementation can prevent or delay its onset. I recommend between 800 and 1200 IU of vitamin E daily for the diabetic.

You may also try adding 200 micrograms of chromium picolinate supplement to your daily diet. It will help your body metabolize carbohydrates, fats, and proteins, controlling the glycosylation. And, as an added bonus, it may increase energy and suppress appetite.

SORBITOL

Sorbitol has become an important matter of discussion because of its use as a popular artificial sweetener. It is allegedly safer than others, but I haven't seen any literature on how the body handles it. What I do know is that natural sorbitol, created in the body, can be a problem for diabetics. If you have diabetes and want to eat or drink a product containing sorbitol, I advise you to talk with your doctor to be certain it is safe for you.

Note: I cannot recommend any artificial sweetener at this time. In the past, every one of them—saccharin, aspartame, sorbitol—has proved to be dangerous for some people. They may even prove more harmful to you than sugar in its many forms— fructose, sucrose, corn syrup, and the like. What the manufacturers of many products don't say is that they use artificial sweeteners to save money.

The one exception, and it is so new to me at this writing that I can't be certain, though I'm currently using it at home, is a product called Stevia. It comes from a South American and Chinese herb and seems both effective and healthy. Only time will tell for certain, though this may be one answer for those who crave sweets.

Another option is to spend some time browsing through some of the excellent cookbooks featuring desserts for diabetics. These recipes feature natural sweeteners—honey, a syrup made from raisins soaked in water, finely chopped carrots, and other safe foods. In this way you can enjoy cakes, cookies, and pies, as well as a variety of beverages and frozen desserts. Some bakeries and large supermarkets even carry commercial products made in this manner. I strongly urge everyone to explore these options, because what is good for a diabetic to eat is good for us all.

Natural sorbitol is formed within your cells through the enzyme aldose reductase. It is a by-product of glucose metabolism, and in a healthy individual it is broken down into fructose, a simple sugar found in some fruit, which is then eliminated from the cell. Diabetics cannot handle sorbitol; for them, the sorbitol-fructose reaction does not take place as it should. Instead, sorbitol accumulates in their bodies and becomes a factor in the debilitating side effects often seen with diabetes.

Sorbitol causes the cells to lose vitamin C, amino acids,

potassium, and some of the B-complex vitamins. And the accumulation of sorbitol in the cells contributes to problems with the nerves, the pancreas, and other parts of the body.

This phenomenon of elevated abnormal blood sugar tends to lead to the phenomenon known as glycosylation. When this occurs, the glucose binds to proteins, causing changes in the structure and function of your body's proteins. These abnormal proteins in the body are factors for the diabetic, affecting the lens of the eye, the myelin sheath surrounding the cells of the nervous system, and the proteins of the red blood cells. They also appear to promote aging for everyone.

Of the drugs frequently prescribed for diabetics to counter the sorbitol problem, all have potential side effects and may ultimately be as much a concern as the reason they were suggested in the first place.

By contrast, an increase in vitamin C has been shown in repeated studies to be more effective than pharmaceuticals in reducing sorbitol levels. It has no side effects, no long-term dangers.

HEART DISEASE

The high rate of heart disease in the United States is the consequence of many aspects of our lives, including our relatively sedentary habits, our consumption of high-fat foods, and our exposure to cigarette smoke and numerous other factors. I will discuss some of these issues in the next chapter, but for now the most important thing to know is that the best natural remedy you can take to combat all of these troubles is a combination of vitamins E and C.

Tobacco smoke has been a trigger for cardiovascular disease throughout the last century. Although tobacco has been used for centuries, cigarette smoking did not begin until well after the Civil War. At that time the Duke family of Durham, North Carolina, and some others found that they could get rich by encouraging the new fad. This was also the time when advertising became more sophisticated, and soon cigarette smoking was being promoted for several purposes. According to the ads, it was good for your health, because it helped you relax and it kept you from overindulging in sweets. It was a refresher, because the nicotine "hit" to the brain brought new energy. It was a social activity. And when movies became popular, it played a major role in seduction. Couples smoked when they met. Couples smoked during verbal foreplay. And couples smoked while basking in the afterglow of intimate relations. The fact that, as early as the 1890s, doctors were finding that people who smoked had a higher risk of heart disease and cancer than non-smokers did nothing to change the attitudes of popular culture. Today, cigarette smoking is still promoted for its sensuality and its ability to enhance or adorn both the smoker's personality and his or her personal life.

But no matter how it is promoted, the inescapable truth is that tobacco smoke contains approximately four thousand chemicals. You ingest them when you smoke. And you ingest them when there's cigarette smoke in the air. No matter how you're exposed to them, the chemicals all attack you in the same manner: They are carried in the bloodstream on the molecules of low-density lipoproteins (LDL), the "bad" cholesterol you hear about, causing oxidative damage to those molecules transporting them and to the arteries. Nor is the damage from smoking limited to the arteries. High blood pressure is increased by smoking. The liver is damaged in such a way that it cannot properly regulate your cholesterol level. The list goes on and on. The hazards for nonsmokers exposed to secondhand smoke are more severe than most people know: More than thirty-seven thousand people die each year from heart disease related directly to secondhand smoke.

One reason it has taken this long for the backlash against smoking to have some measurable effect is that provable knowledge has only recently been found in the results of studies begun just after World War II. One example, a study in England, has followed four thousand children born in 1945 over the last fifty years. It was from these children that we learned pulmonary diseases that occur when people are in their twenties—asthma, chronic bronchitis, etc.—are directly related to lung problems that first cropped up when they were eighteen months to two years old. The young adult onset of the problems was traced to pneumonia and other lung ailments in infancy. In many cases these ailments resulted from mothers who smoked during pregnancy or from an exposure to secondhand smoke when they were newborns. What people did not realize at the time was that giving up smoking is vitally important to having a healthy baby, and that giving it up entirely is the only way to ensure that an infant is not exposed to secondhand smoke. As a result, many of the children raised in the 1940s and 1950s who lived in homes where cigarette smoke constantly hung in the air are now paying for it with their health.

Also, the problems posed from allowing smoking on airplanes were not understood until flight attendants began having lengthy careers. For many years a flight attendant had to be an attractive single female. The earliest ones were registered nurses, though this requirement was later dropped. There were no males. There were no married women. The attendants, though they were really rescue specialists assigned to the planes in case their skills were needed during a crash, became "sky bunnies" in the minds of the mostly male business travelers. The women were highly intelligent, but most looked on their brief flight-attendant career as a way to travel the world, meet men, and eventually get married.

Today there is no such discrimination. Flight attendants are male and female, young and old, frequently married and career-oriented. Many of them have been with the airlines for ten years, twenty years, or longer. And because of their prolonged time in the air, their exposure to the foul, badly recycled air, the secondhand cigarette smoke of the past, and the radiation inherent in high-altitude flying, their bodies have been damaged. In many cases, you can see the accelerated aging process in the faces of flight attendants. You can also now read that their unions are fighting the airlines, because these attendants have a higher incidence of cancer and heart disease than other people their age with similar family histories.

It takes time to prove a theory, and most people will not give up what they consider a pleasure until they feel there is adequate proof of danger.

Today we know that the antioxidant benefits of vitamins C and E are critical for fighting secondhand smoke damage. Thus, even the most health-conscious must take daily supplements to reduce the risk of cardiovascular problems from sources outside their control.

CHOLESTEROL

Cholesterol can be compared with an angry teenager who is having a feud with a kid who lives across town. He has no driver's license, and his parents won't take him where he wants to go, because they know he's going to pick a fight. Instead, he goes out to see if he can hitch a ride. If he can, there will be violence. If he can't, he'll stay at home out of harm's way, sulking but not giving anyone trouble.

Cholesterol is a fat that wants to create havoc by traveling from your liver to your body cells. The only way it can do so is by hitching a ride with the lipoproteins. There are, however, good lipoproteins and bad lipoproteins. Just as the teenager might get picked up by a law enforcement officer, member of the clergy, or someone else who'll help keep him away from trouble, so the potential for physiological "violence" by cholesterol is determined by the lipoproteins.

High-density lipoproteins (HDL) are the do-gooders of the body. They give the cholesterol a ride through the bloodstream, and then take the fat back to the liver, where it's not going to act out against the human in whom it's been traveling.

By contrast, low-density lipoproteins (LDL) are enablers. They like the wild life. They give no thought to the health of the body, and they let the cholesterol travel with them into your cells, where they add to your risk of atherosclerosis.

Vitamin E acts as an undercover officer, hiding in the cells, waiting for the trouble that occurs when LDL is back in town. It enters the cells, where it works to stop the free radical damage. It also increases HDL levels, speeds up the destruction of the protein fibrin, which leads to dangerous clot formation, and serves other protective functions as well.

Tests for the degree of susceptibility to cardiovascular disease have shown that if someone's blood has a high level of vitamin E, he's far less likely to develop cardiovascular problems than someone with a low level. In addition, it appears that when you have a high vitamin E level in the bloodstream, the chance that you may have a stroke is lowered, even if such things as high fat and cholesterol levels might indicate a problem. For those who have already experienced heart disease and/ or stroke, I recommend 3000 to 5000 milligrams of vitamin C and 800 IU to 1200 IU of vitamin E daily.

As with vitamin C and smoking, this does not mean you can indulge in a fast-food diet, popping extra vitamin E just before you reach for the super-giant fries. But it does show that vitamin E, like vitamin C, can assure you better health than your other dietary habits might indicate. And when you put them all together—a change to proper diet coupled with the appropriate supplements—you will prolong your good health and possibly your allotted time on Earth.

Chapter Nine

PUTTING IT ALL
TOGETHER

NOW THAT YOU KNOW about the ten natural remedies that can save your life, I'd like to take you a step further. I want to help you develop a lifestyle that will keep you well if you're healthy, make you well if you're not, and, I hope, ensure that you will never need the natural remedies in this book for a serious illness. If it's too late to avoid health problems, I want to show you how to slow the onset or the progress of potentially debilitating conditions.

Do you remember the quiz I gave you in Chapter 1? Now that you've learned about these ten natural remedies and are ready to apply your new knowledge, I'd like to go over the quiz again.

1. Do you get outside for exercise, like a brisk walk, at least twenty minutes a day, every day? Do you do this during the daylight hours, regardless of the weather?

Exercise is essential for your health. The best exercise puts your lungs and cardiovascular system to work for at least twenty minutes every day. The least expensive form of such exercise is taking a brisk walk, as rapidly as you can while still being comfortable. As your stamina rises, you may choose to increase your pace and your distance.

The reason for doing this is that daylight causes a natural tranquilizer to be produced in your body. Your mind becomes clear and you'll be able to work more effectively when you return.

I recommend such exercise even on stormy days. If that's not realistic, consider indoor options, like climbing stairs or walking around a mall, making sure you have bright full-spectrum light in the places where you can control it.

2. Does your lighting come from standard fluorescent bulbs? Incandescent lamps? Full-spectrum fluorescents?

Full-spectrum light is necessary for your emotional health. It affects the pineal gland, which regulates a number of hormones, including melatonin. This is one of the hormones responsible for your moods. If you stay indoors during most daylight hours, you'll feel depressed even on the nicest of days. A full-spectrum fluorescent bulb that has a rating of 6000 to 6500 degrees Kelvin (which is how lighting is measured) is ideal. This is the same as the midday sun. The lower the number of degrees, the less the amount of good light, the kind that benefits your health.

I recommend that you replace fluorescent bulbs with full-spectrum bulbs. The names vary. You can buy this type of lightbulb at nurseries, garden centers, and lighting stores; these businesses will have catalogs listing the different brands and their Kelvin ratings.

3. Do you eat fast foods, fried foods, or high-sugar foods (like most commercial cereals, as well as pastries and doughnuts) at least three to five times a week or more?

In addition to increasing the possibility of weight gain, such a diet causes nutritional deficiencies. You'll probably get frequent colds throughout the winter, be more susceptible to flu and pneumonia, and have a depressed immune system. The consumption of refined sugar causes your blood sugar to peak and dip. There will be times when you can think clearly and other times when you're so tired that work, play, or anything else seems a chore.

4. Do you eat sweets (including ice cream) as snacks, dessert, or with some frequency?

See the answer to number 3 and add cardiovascular problems. Whole foods contain all the nutrients you need for full metabolization. Processed foods require extra nutrients to keep them from "robbing" what's in your body. All forms of refined sugar require the B-complex vitamins for metabolization, and the easiest way for the body to find these vitamins is to "rob" them from your heart. The heart attack susceptibility of overweight men in their forties is less the result of obesity than it is of malnutrition, caused by the vitamins having to handle the high-sugar diet.

5. Do you find that caffeine doesn't affect you very much? Even if it gives you a lift in the morning and midafternoon, have you noticed that it doesn't interfere with your ability to sleep?

Hypoglycemics find that caffeine doesn't give them the "jolt" they desire; instead, it creates a sugar-adrenaline reaction that makes sleep critical. This is made worse if they combine a cup of coffee with a candy bar, brownie, doughnut, or other high-sugar snack. Whether or not you are hypoglycemic, if you experience these reactions, or want to avoid them, eliminate caffeine from your diet.

6. Do you drink tap water? If you do, whether at home or on the job, do you know whether the pipes that deliver it are made of copper?

Old copper pipes add trace amounts of copper to the water you drink. Although copper is an important mineral, an excess of it can cause a psychological problem often mistaken for mental illness. So if you find you are depressed, and can't pinpoint a valid reason, reach for steam-distilled water for drinking and cooking. It will aid in the excretion of copper and other toxic metals, like lead.

7. Do you drink water to quench your thirst or does much of your liquid come from juice, tea, coffee, and the like?

Your body needs water, not just liquids. As many as eight eight-ounce glasses are critical. You should increase that amount as you get older. I recommend that you drink distilled water. Other liquids are needed in addition, though some, such as caffeinated beverages, can lead to increased urination, which can cause dehydration. So drink more water, not more coffee.

8. Do you engage in any social activity, like bowling, participating in a religious group, playing on a sports team, belonging to a club or fraternal order?

Your long-term physical health will, in large part, be determined by your sense of being part of a caring community. Religious organizations are the ideal, because they're structured around mutual caring. But even regular bowling games with friends can supply the socialization needed for health.

9. Are you in a committed relationship with another person? If not, are you seeking one, or are you just enjoying the casual lifestyle of "playing the field"?

Loners, no matter how well they eat, no matter how many recommended nutritional supplements they take, no matter how much exercise and rest they get, will not have the quality of life of those in committed relationships. To love and be loved, both in an intimate relationship and in the community described in number 8, is to ensure the greatest chance for a long and healthy life.

10. Do you have to travel much by air?

Air travel can cause several problems. First, much of the air is recycled, which increases its carbon dioxide content. In addition, this recycling of airborne organisms can spread the contagious diseases of any passenger. If your immune system is not strong, you may come down with at least a minor cold within a few days of an air trip.

Air travel also exacerbates blood-sugar changes, so the pressurization of the cabin air creates problems for hypoglycemics and diabetics. The rapid change in altitude causes the body to react as though it has had an infusion of sugar. More insulin is needed to metabolize food in the air than is needed on the ground. Air travel will also increase the effect of alcohol. You can get drunk in the air with the same number of drinks that you can consume on the ground without losing control. As a result, my recommendation for those who frequently travel by air is to drink a lot of water to hydrate the body and keep flushing out the system and to be sure to take their vitamin supplements.

11. Do you have to travel in a way that requires you to change one or more time zones?

Time changes affect your biorhythm and ability to sleep, and weaken your immune system. The use of melatonin at these times can help you to rest your body's clock, and vitamins C, E, and B complex will help to handle stress.

12. Do you use a computer at work? At home? Both?

Computer use can limit your exposure to bright light, a major cause of depression and minor sleep disorders. It also limits your physical activity. And it can lead you to develop a casual attitude toward your diet. You can become so engrossed in what you're doing that you forget to eat, or you eat whatever is handy, regardless of its nutritional value. Daylight fluorescent or full-spectrum incandescent lighting should surround you when you work at the computer. Be sure to take frequent breaks for exercise. Watch your diet. And be certain to look away from the screen periodically, focusing on objects at several distances in order to exercise your eye muscles.

13. Do you relax with television or a computer?

This creates the same problem mentioned in number 12. The lack of light often leads to depression, which makes you draw inward, avoiding person-to-person socialization, which leads to still deeper depression. In addition, much of the programming on television is not realistic at best, and violent at worst, which can affect your perception of the world around you.

14. Does your work schedule require you to commute before the sun is fully up or after it has set?

Are you getting the message that light is important? Depression is rapidly becoming the leading problem for which men and women in their most productive years are seeking medical help. This is great for the manufacturers of Prozac and similar drugs. What many people don't realize is that, in many cases, the problem can be their lifestyle, not something wrong with their mind. They're not depressed because of health reasons. They're depressed because of the lack of light. As I've said before, be sure to get outside for regular "light" breaks during the day if your schedule does not allow you to spend time in the sun in the morning and afternoon.

15. Do you work irregular shifts on your job—first shift one week and third shift another?

Your body needs to be stabilized for quality sleep. Maybe you can't avoid these shift changes, but you can turn night into day and day into night. Be certain to use very bright lights when you're up, and then dim them greatly, and take melatonin, before you go to sleep. Use blackout curtains or a sleep mask to make your bedroom seem to be in the middle of night. Recognize that you'll be under a constant stress until you can stabilize your work-sleep time. Melatonin and stress-related vitamins such as B complex, C, and E are extremely useful.

16. Do you work the third shift, coming home when others are waking up and preparing to go to work?

You must be sure to create a light-dark arrangement that matches what you'd experience if you worked the first shift. Follow the procedures listed in number 15. The only difference is that with the stability of third-shift work, you shouldn't need extra vitamins.

17. Do you smoke?

You already know about the problems caused by nicotine: how it increases the risk of a number of cancers. In addition, smokers also have a problem with hypoglycemia, and because cigarette tobacco is sugar-cured, that makes smoke more of a problem than candy. Hypoglycemia can also help cause depression, especially if you drink beverages with caffeine. All three substances—nicotine, sugar, and caffeine—cause wide swings in blood sugar. These adversely affect brain function and lead to mood swings.

18. Do you live with a smoker or work where you're exposed to cigarette, pipe, or cigar smoke?

See the preceding answer. The biggest difference is that when you experience mild depression, you probably won't connect it to the secondhand smoke. This is yet another reason why so many people are taking the milder antidepressant drugs when they don't need them. Instead, I recommend you increase your daily intake of antioxidant vitamins to 3000 milligrams to 6000 milligrams of vitamin C and 800 to 1200 IU of vitamin E.

19. Do you take any form of nutritional supplement?

Nutritional supplements can counter a multitude of environmental problems and personal "sins." You've already taken a first step toward reversing degenerative disease, immune system malfunction, and other problems for your body.

20. Do you cook for yourself or rely on packaged foods you only have to heat and serve?

The quality of your food, the dangers of your reacting to preservatives, food coloring, and various additives, and your need for nutritional supplements are all determined by the way you prepare meals. Allergic reactions, immune system disorders, fatigue, and depression can be triggered by the food you eat. My recommendation is to eat as little prepared and prepackaged food as possible, and to get a minimum of five servings of fruit and vegetables each day and two servings of fish a week.

21. Do you eat beef? Pork? Chicken? Turkey? Fish?

Every food has its value and its risk. Beef is not good for our cardiovascular systems, and the way the animals have been fed has occasionally led to such scandals as the "mad cow" disease. Chickens are often given hormones, meant to spur growth. Many chicken farms don't allow the birds to move out of multi-tiered cages. That may speed their growth, but it creates unhealthy birds. And that can affect the eater. Fish carry the toxic metals that pollute our waters unless they're raised carefully in controlled circumstances or regularly checked in the wild. And so it goes. The more you learn about the animals and the conditions under which they're raised, the better your judgment call will be. Our bodies are biochemically able to digest meat, yet the type of meat and the way it's raised are concerns for all of us.

22. Are you a vegetarian? Do you rely on a variety of vegetarian protein sources for the full range of protein your body needs?

Unknowledgeable vegetarians are often malnourished. We humans are omnivores who do not need to eat meat when we consume that right blend of protein in our diet. A vegetarian diet based on full understanding of your body's needs can be very healthful. Without that knowledge and effort, you're going to be no healthier than the person who delights in beef rippled with fat as his primary source of nutrition.

23. Do you work or live in a building that recirculates the air, or do you have a source of continuous fresh air, perhaps through open windows?

Newer buildings designed for efficiency often don't have windows that open. Spores, bacteria, and other dangers lurk in uncleaned air-recycling systems, even when the air itself is supposedly cleaned. These closed heating and cooling systems have also been the source of illness. All such systems may lower the immune system while exposing you to a variety of contagious diseases. Again, outdoor fresh air and light breaks are necessary for your good health, as are antioxidant vitamin supplements.

24. Are you able to sleep through the night, or do you have interruptions—from small children, a sick family member, or someone else?

The lack of sleep has a negative effect on your immune system and may be a cause of depression. People who know their sleep will be interrupted should use supplements and be careful that their diet and exercise schedule keeps their resistance as high as possible.

25. Do you drink alcoholic beverages or regular soft drinks?

The sugar in these beverages will lead to hypoglycemic reactions, depression, and a depressed immune system. This doesn't mean you can never have them. Moderate use, however, carries with it the responsibility to use your supplements, to exercise, and to take antistress vitamins. These may help you handle the problems caused by alcohol and sugared beverages.

Now that you've assessed your personal situation in light of your new knowledge, and are considering the possibility of making some dietary and lifestyle changes, it's time to discuss how you can fight conditions that have never before existed or have never before been so pervasive in society. In recent years, we've made remarkable progress in our medical knowledge, but we've fallen far behind in our ability to deal with the dangers posed by advances in technology.

If you were born shortly after World War II, within your lifetime you've had to deal with the nutritional deficiencies of TV dinners and the electromagnetic-radiation dangers of electric blankets, television sets, and computer monitors. You've suffered the buildup of bacteria and other biological "bad guys" in the heating and cooling systems of sealed office buildings. You've experienced new allergens in the latest materials used in, for example, carpet backing. You've seen phosphates put into laundry detergents, fluoride added to drinking water, insecticides placed on just about anything that grows, hormones mixed into animal feed, and radiation used to prolong the shelf life of milk and other products. Yet modern medicine has continued to respond only to the illnesses of your parents, grandparents, and great-grandparents, depending on your age. Natural remedies are the quickest, most effective way to combat these new factors and help you thrive in the years to come.

I want to address the baby boomers first. Yours was the transitional generation, not because it was so large but because it was the first group in American history to elevate science to godlike status. You were taught to accept new technology without questioning it. You were taught to embrace the unproven, to seek shortcuts without looking for hidden pitfalls. As a result, your lives have been altered, and the lives of succeeding generations will be altered, in ways that sometimes lead us from the light back into the darkness.

If we can date the time when the best of intentions became the first few steps along the footpath to the Hell of premature aging and death, it would be the end of World War II. The effort by the Allies to fight the Axis powers led to accelerated research and development in everything from weapons to air-

craft, pharmaceuticals to surgery. What had originally been created for the purpose of either destroying enemy strongholds or
saving the lives of the Allies was often found to have peacetime
applications. Advances in airline technology, new forms of
communication, and many other good things came out of the
race to outwit the enemy. In fact, so different, so much easier
did life become that every discovery was hailed as an advance.
Only later did we learn how foolish was our thinking. It is only
now that we are beginning to understand what this has done to
our health and the health of our children.

The problem originates with the American desire for
change. If we read about new discoveries that sound helpful, we
want to use them instantly. We know we are technologically
blessed and consider it the height of sophistication if we rush to
embrace each new wonder of the scientist's laboratory.

If you were growing up in the 1950s, for example, and
needed a new pair of shoes, there was a good chance that your
shoe store had what was called a fluoroscope. It was a kid-sized
variation of the medical fluoroscope, a device used by physicians in the 1920s to 1930s to give a quick X ray–type view of
part of a patient's body. At the bottom of the box was a hole
into which you'd place your feet, side by side. Then you'd look
down and, wonder of wonders, you could see the skeletal structure of your feet in the new shoes your parents were planning to
buy you. The store clerk had already measured the length and
width of your feet. You'd already tried on the shoes. You'd
walked around a little to "see how they feel." But then, just
before you were given your free comic book, you got to see how
great the fit was in the marvelous fluoroscope. In fact, if you'd
been rowdy and had a sibling still in need of shoes, you might
have been encouraged to linger, because the fun of watching
yourself wiggle your toes was keeping you quiet, and the shop-

keeper was anxious to make the trip easier on your parents so that they'd buy more shoes.

And what did the fluoroscope really do for you? It exposed you to doses of poorly shielded radiation.

Radiation is cumulative. All the radiation to which you are exposed in your lifetime, from sunshine to dental X rays, lingers in your body. That use of the fluoroscope was like adding gunpowder to an explosive. A little gunpowder can make a firecracker. A lot of gunpowder can make a bomb capable of destroying a portion of a city. Depending on your exposures since childhood, that fluoroscope exposure could prove to be a health threat now or in the years to come.

In past generations, most people were not as affected by radiation as they are today. Agricultural workers learned to wear long-sleeved shirts and wide-brimmed hats to avoid forms of skin cancer. The average person rarely had X rays; usually it was a once-in-a-lifetime experience. But the baby boomers got to take advantage of the new technology. Dentists would X ray their teeth at every visit, the equipment often "leaking" radiation, compared with the pinpoint accuracy of the latest equipment. Hospitals would sometimes take X rays every time a parent brought in a child who'd fallen and hurt herself, even when the doctor had determined nothing was broken. ("Better to be safe than sorry, and the hospital has this new, state-of-the-art equipment . . .") Wristwatches had the numbers painted with radioactive paint so that the watch would glow in the dark, allowing you to know the time in the middle of the night. And fluoroscopes helped you see your feet as you wiggled them in your shoes.

Science marched on!

Then there were the insects. A number of cities, and the wealthier and more desirable suburbs, decided that God made a mistake in creating mosquitoes and other pests. Through the wonders of science, namely, insecticides like DDT, nature could be changed for the better. And so, throughout the spring and summer months, there would be periodic warnings to stay inside your house for a few minutes at an early hour of the morning.

At the appointed time, a truck with a massive sprayer would lumber down the street. The trees would be covered with chemicals that would drip down like rain long after the spraying was completed. The liquid would land on the grass, get into the soil, and frequently drip on schoolchildren heading for classes.

No one thought anything of it. The days would be free from many of the insects the residents hated. Mosquito bites would be down, rosebushes were likely to bloom without being eaten, and gardens would thrive, the harmful "bugs" having been banished through the wonders of science.

Remember our discussion of DES (diethylstilbestrol) in Chapter 7? It was the wonder drug, introduced in 1945, that was supposed to help bring high-risk babies to term. That concept is not gone from modern thinking. We don't feed cows DES with their food, but we do give them other hormone products that are passed on to the consumer. Growth hormone, a potentially dangerous substance, and synthetic estrogens are classic examples.

What does this mean today? No one is certain. What we do know is that milk consumption has been on the rise for many years, that hormone-fed animal and milk products have become a large part of our diets, and that during this same period, estrogen levels have increased and testosterone levels have decreased.

The testosterone issue is an interesting one, due to another statistic: Violence among younger males has been on the rise in recent years. Schoolyard battles, bar fights, domestic violence, dangerously aggressive driving ("road rage"), and the like are all on an increase. Sociologists like to blame such horrors on popular culture—music lyrics favoring violence; action-adventure movies in which manliness is determined by fists, guns, knives, and bombs; and video games in which a win is a kill. All these factors are undoubtedly important, but my assertion is that the reduction in testosterone is at least as critical. This is especially true since males exposed to the same popular culture influences who did not exhibit the same extreme behavior had higher levels of testosterone.

As was mentioned in Chapter 7, thalidomide had a shameful history beginning at about the same time DES was being prescribed. This was another drug meant to help pregnant mothers. Instead, it caused birth defects in many of their babies, terrible defects. A child might be born with arms missing the bone from the elbow to the wrist. Or she would have hands attached right at the elbow. Another child might be born a torso and a head, missing arms and legs. These children were not mentally damaged, unless you consider the psychological problems of their going through life as they had to. They often had the intelligence to be doctors, inventors, scientists, teachers, and anything else they might desire. Tragically, for some the handicaps were too great to overcome.

The question about thalidomide that has not yet been answered is whether the survivors, many of whom are now adults, will have genetically damaged children. And if their children are normal in appearance, is there a genetic time bomb that will skip a generation before exploding?

Other advances have created unknown problems. Electric blankets came into use for the baby boomers, and many of these blankets, especially the early ones, are suspected of having caused long-term health consequences due to the electromagnetic field to which they exposed their users.

The early microwave ovens often had leaky gasket seals. You could detect the problem by running your finger around the rubber while the microwave was working. If you got a tiny burn, you knew it needed to go to the shop. What was not said was that your exposure to the leak while you worked in the kitchen might damage your eyes.

Television sets, both black-and-white and color, were considered dangerous leakers of radiation. Schoolteachers taught their students that it was unhealthy to sit closer than three or four feet from the set, and sitting at least six feet away was better. But the sets were costly, so most people bought small screens. And kids being kids, there was a tendency among them to sit almost on top of the sets.

The radiation danger from computer monitors was so great in early models that companies developed shields you could buy. Studies in Canada led that country's postal system, which includes its telephone company, to ban pregnant women from computer jobs until after they had given birth. Such precautions, however, were rarely taken in the United States.

The lead used in gasolines became a concern when the interstate highway system was developed, car prices were reduced, and people drove everywhere. In this way, pollution was added to the problems created by an increasingly sedentary lifestyle.

Then there are the drugs, the "uppers" and "downers" seen as the answer to everyone's busy work schedules. It was 1938 when amphetamines became America's wonder drug, a role they would play for more than twenty-five years. They were untested, of course. They had met the general standards to allow their sale, but, as is too often the case, no one understood the full implications of amphetamine use. Or the implications of amphetamines being combined with the equally "safe" phenobarbitol.

For the next quarter century, the public delighted in these wonderful pills. They curbed your appetite and gave you greater energy, allowing weight loss and productivity. What no one talked about was their addictive nature, or that the nation was changing its ideal of beauty from a normal woman, with a less-than-"perfect" figure, to the ultra-thin anomaly of the "super model." These pills helped women achieve the desired thinness, and so pervasive did the "need" become that, by the time the baby boomers were being born, in 1946, their mothers and fathers considered the pills a normal part of the day's health regimen. By the 1960s, when the dangers were understood and the use of these pills declined, the new "perfect" figure for women was so popular that medication was replaced with the unending diet regimes and—at the extreme—anorexia nervosa and bulimia, which still constitute "eating" for thousands of women today.

The most public display of this problem occurred at MGM studios during the period when child stars like Judy Garland were working there. In 1969, Judy Garland accidentally overdosed on the drugs the studio had been giving her since she was a teenager. She is often seen as an anomaly, unrelated to the greater context of the problem. But the truth is that almost everyone in the studio took the drugs, including Louis B. Mayer. The personnel were monitored by the studio physician. He, in turn, had as little knowledge of the potential problems as the innocent public, misled by "science" about the effects.

Sleeping pills were soon added to this inventory. Many people took a stimulant to wake up in the morning and a sleeping pill at night. In fact, if you watch television shows and movies from the 1950s, you'll see how pervasive it became. It was common to hear dialogue in which someone was told to take a "diet pill" or a "wake-up pill." Or to hear someone suggest that the heroine take a sleeping pill to ensure a good night's rest. These pills were mainstream, and it was no more shocking than if a character in a contemporary film said, "Don't forget to take your vitamins."

We did not know, of course, that the stimulants could lead to malnutrition, organ damage, and chemical dependency, and that sleeping pills should have been classed as knockout drops. What was never discussed was that there are different levels of sleep in a normal night, and sleeping pills render a person unconscious without letting them reach the deepest level of sleep. That deepest level is where real rest comes, where the body heals itself and the mind sometimes vents the pressures of the day through dreams. We now know that a person who regularly uses sleeping pills and remains unconscious in bed for eight hours a night will be far less rested, and certainly less healthy, than someone who gets only six hours of natural sleep a night. This is not to say that six hours is adequate sleep—it is not for most people—but natural sleep takes you through all the stages of rest. Sleeping pills do not allow this.

The result was a growing number of "zombies"—"walking dead." They were always tired, always malnourished, and always certain everything was fine, just fine. They had energy. They had stamina. They had heart attacks. They had kidney damage.

You get the picture. And from the drug addictions inadvertently foisted on the baby boomers we have grown into a nation that runs on Valium, Prozac, and every other pharmaceutical flavor of the month, all to the detriment of our bodies.

(Brief history lesson. It was not until 1982 that the Betty Ford Clinic was opened in California. Many treatment facilities existed before then, and many wealthy and well-known people were quietly going to them. But until Betty Ford, addiction meant an inner-city derelict, a poorly educated, hopelessly pathetic person with a wasted life. The few "nice" people who spoke of addiction were treated as tragic aberrations. They had somehow managed to fall among the lowlifes, and it was only because they were "better" than the others that there was hope for them. Betty Ford made people realize that addiction was everyone's concern. It was only then that we as a culture began thinking that an alternative to pharmaceuticals might be good.)

Unfortunately, our newfound awareness is limited. Americans tend to focus their fears of addiction on a single drug at a time. This one is bad. That one, just introduced by an enlightened research team, is good. We feel safe in adopting the new, when, in fact, all we may be doing is falling into another trap.

Many baby boomers were children when TV dinners were introduced to the world. Television was a curiosity that many families chose to be part of their lifestyle. In these homes, the children arrived home from school between 3:30 and 4 P.M. They were given their snack of milk and cookies, and, by five o'clock, were placed in front of the television set for an hour of programs aimed especially at them. These had to do with Howdy Doody, America's most popular puppet show, or one of the Western series, starring Wild Bill Hickok or Roy Rogers and Dale Evans. Then at 6 P.M. came the news. At that point, the family would sit at the dinner table, place the television, if it was movable, where everyone could see it, and watch the events of the day as told to them by the newscaster.

Since many televisions were console models, even if their screens were small, it became more convenient to eat in the room where the television was part of the furniture. First came folding trays to use to hold the food. And then came TV dinners.

The nutritional value of TV dinners was like that of many of the breakfast cereals advertised on TV. There was probably as much nourishment in them as in the packaging.

The main portions of the TV dinner varied, but they were always high in starch. There may have been small pieces of fried chicken, heavily coated with some substance that tasted delicious when hot but congealed into goo when it cooled on the chicken. There may have been turkey or meat loaf, perhaps with corn or peas; mashed potatoes were frequently on hand. Many of the packages had a dessert of one sort or another, and all had the attraction of needing only to be taken from the freezer, heated in the oven, and placed on the tray, once the covering foil was removed. Add milk or coffee, and you had a complete meal.

The popularity of these meals became evident in the private lives of the rich and famous. The late Cary Grant was an actor who epitomized sophistication on the screen. When he invited the equally suave, handsome, and sophisticated actor Peter Lawford to dinner, he brought out tray tables and TV dinners. That was the effect those nonnutritious time-savers had on American culture.

Then there was the typical American work week. Parents of the baby boomers who were in the forefront of union activity fought hard to win a five-day, forty-hour work week for everyone. Laborers benefited and so did management, and weekends became family times. Stores that were open on weekends tried to arrange for the single members of their staffs to work on those days if possible. Only rarely did you find late-night closings on the weekends. In fact, in many instances, department stores would close at 5 or 5:30 P.M. on Friday and Saturday, and then be closed on Sunday. There would be one or two late nights during the week; "late" would mean 8 P.M.

Today many supermarkets operate twenty-four hours a day, convenience food stores are open for eighteen or more hours a day, drugstores have twenty-four-hour drive-through windows, fast-food restaurants may be open as late as 3 or 4 A.M., and department stores in malls may consider 10 P.M. an early closing. Only hourly workers, like restaurant personnel, are likely to be asked to work fewer than forty hours, and that's so that management can avoid paying for benefits. The managers, however, who work on salary, are usually assigned a forty-eight-hour or a fifty-hour work week.

Law offices burn the midnight oil. Some HMOs demand that many of their offices keep hours similar to those of hospital emergency rooms, making them available to the public as much as sixteen hours a day. The rise of relatively inexpensive computers with modem links to home offices anywhere in the world has led some companies to assign workloads that cannot be completed on the job. Instead, employees are expected to use the various linking systems, from e-mail to sophisticated Internet connections, to finish at home what once would have been accomplished in the office. We have forgotten how to rest.

In contrast, nineteenth-century agricultural workers, laboring with hand tools, simple mechanical devices, and horsepower, did not, in many cases, work as hard as some office workers. The farm life may have been physically demanding, but the long hours were seasonal. There was a time to clear, to sow, to nurture, to harvest, and to rest. The year had a rhythm that made for a healthier life than the intensely pressured existence brought to us by labor-saving devices such as the computer. And any work on Sunday was strictly forbidden.

When we do find time to relax, even our entertainment has become so constricting that we've stopped socializing. Instead, we avoid face-to-face communication by using Internet chat rooms. We don't share an experience in the movie theater as much as we isolate ourselves with VCRs and other forms of home entertainment systems. We don't go to concerts and clubs as much as we buy cassette tapes and CDs. We isolate ourselves from life with Walkman-type players and noise-blocking headphones. We turn our automobiles into rolling isolation booths, cranking up the music, talking on our cell phones, and munching on the carry-out conveniently placed in the cup holder. We live our lives with the windows rolled up, socializing in absentia. We have virtual friends, even though our good health depends on our having real ones.

The fact is, the human body was meant for close interpersonal contact. When we touch a loved one, our blood pressure gets lower, our respiration slows, we become calmer, at peace. This is why couples who have been long married talk of the joy of lying in bed, "snuggling"—holding each other, touching, talking quietly. They are strengthening their relationship, strengthening their immune system, improving their health. The act of intercourse is immensely enjoyable, but it's often secondary to what might be considered foreplay. This actually is the best medicine. It is the gentle physical contact that reminds us that we love and are loved in return.

Popular culture has, for generations, glorified committed love and denounced casual relationships. This was not just because of a puritanical streak. Humans have always sensed what medical research has now proven, that in committed intimacy there is healing, rest, and peace.

Contemporary society adds to its health problems by avoiding that truth. Our actions point toward instant gratification of short-term feelings, not realizing that what is right in a relationship is also necessary for long-term health. Telephone sex via 900 numbers between strangers, casual or close acquaintances, is like using stimulants to wake up in the morning and sleeping pills when going to bed. And if we fail to sustain and build our relationships, we lose the physiological benefits that love brings to the human body.

FOR THOSE WHO MISSED THE BABY BOOM

If you predate the baby boomers, chances are your health is better than theirs, because you were exposed to fewer dangers when you were growing up. You encountered some of the benefits of pharmaceuticals, including the widespread availability of penicillin. But if you're healthy, that's probably because you had a healthy start. Your family may have had a vegetable garden, even if it was one of the Victory Gardens of World War II. You may have been raised in an agricultural area or you may have had relatives who worked on farms and frequently provided your family with free-range meat and poultry and produce that was grown without insecticides.

If you were poor, with a limited variety of food in your diet, there's a good chance that the preparation was healthier than what you'd get in the same circumstances today. Often low income meant a vegetarian diet coupled with fish caught in water not yet poisoned by mercury and other toxic wastes or chickens raised in the backyard.

If you could afford to eat out, you didn't encounter deep-fried, mass-produced food. Maybe you ordered a milk shake, not a nondairy shake, as is served by most fast-food chains. Your bread might have been whole grain, not white bread with twenty or more of the essential nutrients removed with eight, ten, or twelve returned to the bread so that it could be called enriched.

This healthier start will make it easier now for you to regain good health and restore muscle tone, mental alertness, and many of the other indicators of aging you may once have thought unavoidable and irreversible. Instead of being too old to get in the best shape of your life, your age may work to your advantage.

If you are from one of the generations that followed the baby boom, the long-term outlook for your health is still an unknown. You missed some of the dangers your parents unwittingly met, like the fluoroscopes, but you were probably taught that convenience and being happily full were more important than getting proper nutrition. You may be more physically active—and that is important—but you may be carrying a genetic problem as a result of your parents' experiences. In addition, it is likely we will discover as-yet-unknown harm we may have been causing ourselves through the use of many of today's fertilizers, pesticides, pharmaceuticals, and cleaning agents. In fact, on October 5, 1998, the Environmental Protection Agency announced plans to test fifteen thousand chemicals found in a range of products from pesticides to cleansers used around the home. The announcement was mentioned on the inside pages of those newspapers that bothered to report it at all. Most reporters didn't understand the meaning of the announcement; it was an admission that there are problems lurking in chemicals to which we have exposed our families, thinking they were safe.

Ultimately, sixty-two thousand chemicals are to be tested. The first testing will be done on common products that contain potentially toxic chemicals. The EPA is finally acknowledging that, for a long time, large amounts of untested chemicals have been in frequent use. It is good that this initiative has been launched, but by the time all the chemicals have been tested and the results are known, we will have been exposed to them for too many years. The ultimate effect may be any number of health problems we shall have to combat with natural remedies for the rest of our lives.

To add to the horror story, this isn't the first such situation. Many years ago the Environmental Protection Agency put together what it called the GRAS list. It comprised untested products, like aspirin, that had been in use for so long that they were Generally Regarded As Safe. Critics of the GRAS list pointed out that one in four adults has an adverse reaction to aspirin alone! The danger to children from aspirin is even greater. And that's just one of more than four thousand products on the GRAS list. Add the sixty-two thousand chemicals from the current listing, and you get an idea of the scope of the problems we face.

Because of all this, the sooner you develop a proper lifestyle that includes the ten natural remedies that can save your life, the greater your chance of having to face only minimal health problems.

What does this mean for the American culture and many other "advanced" nations? By neglecting to use natural remedies, we've come up with what is literally a sick society. Earlier in the book, we discussed some of the problems with water and air. But in many ways, we've made a lifestyle that works against our health. I am going to suggest a program that takes into account what you've learned so that you can adjust your habits accordingly, and save your life.

STEP 1

Recognize that everything matters. Every decision you make, from the moment you wake until the moment you fall asleep, can affect your health. Humans vary in their needs. One person may find pulsating music relaxing, while his cousin finds it unbearably raucous. You may delight in crowds, whether in shopping malls, nightclubs, or on the city streets, while your neighbor craves the solitude of pastoral settings. You may want a half dozen children, while your brother feels that children would put too much stress on his life. Whatever the case, each of us must find the right lifestyle. But at the same time, we need to recognize that our bodies require daily maintenance in order for us to stay healthy; we have basic needs that must be met, no matter how inconvenient or antithetical to our personality. These include:

1. *Daylight and Exercise.* I don't mean bright, sunny days, though these are ideal times to be out and about. But even if you live in an area that has lots of rain or heavy snow, you still must get outside at least twenty minutes a day. You should supplement this exposure with the use of as much full-spectrum (daylight) light as you can get. Even the artificial light around you should be bright until approximately an hour before you go to bed.

Back in the 1970s, I once knew a police chief in a small community who suffered a heart attack when he was in his early forties. The damage was so considerable that he was forced to retire immediately. His doctor, however, instead of encouraging the patient to rest after an attack that came close to being fatal, told him to walk as briskly as he could for an hour each day. He was to walk in good weather and bad, whether it was warm and sunny or whether he had to bundle up against torrential rain. There were to be no exceptions, no time off.

"But what if I catch pneumonia?" the former chief asked.

"We can treat pneumonia," his doctor responded. "We can't bring you back from the dead."

The physician was heretical for his time. Many doctors of that day would have told the former chief to stay indoors and take up sedentary activities. And he would probably have been dead in three years, based on the post–heart attack survival statistics we have for those days. Getting out and walking each day to strengthen the heart, the lungs, and the body is almost like a resurrection from the dead, because the exercise serves two important purposes.

Exercise strengthens the heart muscles. The cardiovascular strengthening brought about by walking will help make the diseased heart work to its fullest capacity. This knowledge is relatively recent, though we have long-term results from pioneering physicians who defied the conventional wisdom and got their patients moving twenty and twenty-five years ago. In a remarkable number of instances, those patients are still active in their late sixties and seventies, apparently headed for the normal life span once thought impossible. And though some take medication or have other problems, many have done little more than alter their eating and exercise habits.

This simple but effective cardiovascular exercise will, of course, strengthen the healthy person's heart. In fact, if you have a choice between working out in a health spa and walking as rapidly as you can for the same hour you'd spend indoors, try the walk. It is far better for your body. Maybe you won't gain the outward physical appearance you desire. Maybe you won't be able to brag about your personal trainer or attend Christmas parties with those with whom you've shed sweat all year. But you will have maintained excellent cardiovascular fitness without high cost or strenuous effort on high-tech machines.

Always remember that physical fitness was once the natural outcome of ordinary daily activity. People walked to work. They walked to the store. They walked to school. They walked when working in the fields. They walked for companionship. And they combined this natural exercise with the physical labor of growing food, preparing meals, working about the house, growing food, working in manufacturing, and performing their factory jobs. The workout environment of a gym or a health club is a relatively recent phenomenon.

In the 1950s and 1960s gyms were for bodybuilders, weight lifters, and boxers. There were also rooms at places like the YMCA where people could work out on their own. But the idea of a health club as a routine part of the average person's day, or of a fitness center as a corporate perquisite, is new to our society. It's also unnecessary, and increases stress for some people. These are the ones who should get more exposure to daylight, something not possible with the lighting in most clubs, or the ones who are intimidated by the social aspect of the clubs. They become so concerned with how they look and what others think of them that they fail to relax and enjoy all the good they're doing for their bodies.

As I've said before, there is a second element to the daylight walk that fits well within the natural remedies we have discussed. The fact is, a biochemical change takes place when we are exposed to daylight. The sun triggers the release of a natural tranquilizer. This ensures that the walk is calming, that it lowers the blood pressure, strengthens the immune system, and changes your emotional state.

Some psychiatrists working with severely depressed patients now prescribe a daily walk at the start of therapy sessions. They've found that someone who's filled with self-hatred, dissatisfaction, and difficulty in getting through the day may resist talking. This type of patient often feels so terrible about himself that he's afraid of the therapeutic process. He fears he may really be as "bad" as he thinks he is. And while this is never the case—he can always change and live a better life—he's probably not ready to accept that notion. Instead, he goes to the therapist with the expressed or unexpressed idea that, as change cannot occur, he won't commit to more than two or three sessions.

The therapist doesn't try to talk about his problems during their first meeting. Instead, she convinces the new patient to take at least a half hour a day to go for a brisk walk. In every case I've heard about, the patient who heeds the advice starts his second session feeling better than he's felt in months. The improvement is so marked that he's willing to trust the therapist, to be open, to talk freely. He has begun to believe that change may really be possible.

At the same time you're working out your walking schedule, look at the lighting in your home, office, and anywhere else that is within your control. Even in a structured cubicle, perhaps you can add a desk lamp with a daylight fluorescent bulb.

Remember that the brighter you keep your days, the better.

Then, when possible, plan your pre-bedtime activities around a reduction in light, perhaps maybe by getting dimmers for the lights at home.

2. *Diet*. What you eat is a major factor in your health. There are those with lean "hard bodies" whose diets are so poor, their bodies are like poorly made toys. That is, they look great on the outside, but after you use them a few times, they fall apart.

A number of years ago, one of the last of the Fred Harvey Restaurants closed in Cleveland's Terminal Tower. In 1945, the building served the needs of more railroad passengers than any other station in the country, including New York's Grand Central Terminal.

The maître d' of the Fred Harvey facility in Cleveland's Terminal Tower was a man almost as old as the Harvey chain. He eventually retired at the age of 102, and he died three years later. But until he died, he walked to the YMCA, almost twenty blocks from his workplace, and ran the track every day. He considered the handling of loaded trays at the restaurant to be an adequate weight-bearing activity for his body; the walk and run were to handle his cardiovascular requirements.

I mention him because of an incident that occurred when he was in his late nineties. A bodybuilder everyone thought would be the next Mr. Ohio and who was a serious contender for the Mr. America competition did his training at the same YMCA. Each day, the maître d' would watch the man work out, and one day he told the bodybuilder that he was worried about the man's health. He feared that the man, who looked flawlessly sculpted, was a heart attack waiting to happen. To support his hunch, he invited the youth for a jog around the track. The bodybuilder didn't make a quarter of a mile before having chest pains and breathing difficulties. His heart had been weakened by his exercise program, not strengthened as had the maître d's. The bodybuilder was on his way to having the best-looking corpse in the morgue.

He sought the advice of a physician and soon changed his routine. He added walking, then running, and eventually became a champion bodybuilder, with excellent cardiovascular function. Had it not been for the old man, who instinctively understood what was necessary for the human body, he might have died or been crippled from the repetitive stress of his weight lifting.

In the same way, the food you eat—and choose not to eat— can affect you internally long before the results show on the outside. There are people in "glamour" professions—models, actors, dancers—who need to fight to keep their weight down in order to work. This emphasis on being thin is often encouraged by unknowing or unthinking modeling agents, ballet masters, commercial photographers, and casting directors. A number of ballet dancers' memoirs have mentioned the forced change in their eating habits. Women who were beautiful, graceful, and seemingly powerful on the outside were dying on the inside.

In addition to poor or erratic eating habits, concern about physical appearance also leads to self-destructive behavior among many women and some men in the glamour professions. The use of stimulants coupled with alcohol is common. Many people who maintain their weight in such a manner think that drugs and wine form a sociable, "safe" alternative to the eating and purging disorders that were relied on by some models in the past. Anorexia nervosa and bulimia are still matters of concern, and in an effort to be "healthy," many turn back to drugs.

Likewise, there are those who are obese and tackle their problem through what is called yo-yo dieting. They'll use drugs to curb their appetites. Or they'll try fasting. Or they'll get special supplements and drinks that are more chemical than nutritive.

Others seek a healthy approach by joining Overeaters Anonymous or one of the weight-loss programs that relies on changing their eating habits. In this way, they can lose the weight slowly and safely. For many, perhaps most, the weight loss will be permanent. But among those who try this sensible approach, some will again start to eat the wrong foods in the wrong amounts after they've enjoyed their new looks for a while. Their weight will slowly creep back up. At this point, they may repeat the pattern or try a different program. These people go up and down, fat to thin, over and over, like a yo-yo.

We now know that the person who is overweight and takes on a program of positive cardiovascular activities, combined with a healthy diet, will be much healthier and live longer than the yo-yo dieter. The latter creates serious stress on his body, stress that is not magically healed during his periods of thinness. It is actually better to remain at whatever weight you are, as long as you take care of your health in other ways, than to be constantly fluctuating.

I am not going to recommend a specific diet for you. You already know the dangers of a fast-food society. You know that "junk food" got that name for a valid reason. You don't need me to play the role of scolding parent or repeat advice you can find in many newspapers or magazines. Instead, I'm going to emphasize the radical suggestion I made earlier. It will be the first step in maintaining your good health or in restoring your body if you're currently not well. That is, follow a diet that, to a large degree, would be considered appropriate for someone with diabetes.

I know. I've already mentioned this, but I must emphasize the appropriateness of the food choices necessary for everyone. I say this even though I know that many of you may think of it as one of those diets where nothing tastes good, everything is bland, and everything is boring.

First, I don't mean for you to have to have the exact diet as a diabetic seeking to control the condition solely through diet and exercise. But I do expect you to eliminate as much sugar as possible. I do expect you to reduce or eliminate your intake of red meat, poultry fat, and similar substances. And I do expect you to consider, with due seriousness, how to change your meal habits and snacks, though not to the degree you may think.

You already know that one need for healthier eating is fresh fruit and vegetables, something that is critical for diabetics. What you may not realize is that they are important for diabetics for the same reason they are important for your healthier lifestyle.

Apples, bananas, beets, cabbage, citrus fruit, okra, and dried peas all contain pectin, an additive also found in naturally sweetened fruit preserves. Pectin helps to lower cholesterol and to remove metals and toxins from your body. It slows food absorption, and lessens your chance of getting gallstones and heart disease. And if you're being treated for a disease, pectin will help reduce the unpleasant side effects of X rays and radiation therapy.

Pectin is a soluble fiber that makes you feel full, so that you reduce the amount of food you eat, and that's why foods rich in pectin, like apples, are an important part of a weight-loss diet.

Another advantage to soluble natural fiber—you can gain it

by eating a baked potato with its skin on—is that it forms a gel in the small intestines that slows the absorption of glucose. It also slows the time it takes for food to go through your body even while it increases the frequency of your bowel movements. Ultimately it helps to stabilize your blood sugar, reduce gas, and speed up production of bile acid, all improvements for your health.

Ideally, your diet should be based on a low-fat, high-complex-carbohydrate program that will be easy to follow. I don't mean that you should adopt a "deprive yourself and be miserable" regimen. Most people find a new diet more enjoyable than the way they'd been eating before, with the possible exception of the loss of a favorite snack. "How can I give up my delicious candy?" one person will moan. Another may find it hard to give up a favorite layer cake. Still another may think barbecued ribs are a foretaste of the dining table in Heaven. None of these options is a problem if it is an occasional indulgence.

What I ask is that you engage in self-restraint. If you love to have a piece of cake that's made with sugar, do so, but only occasionally. I know a man who loves chocolate-covered raisins, the type you can buy in movie theaters. He used to stock them in a drawer of his desk at work. Now he buys a box only when he goes to see a movie, and since he and his wife are able to take in a new movie only every eight to ten weeks, the occasional indulgence causes him no harm.

Some people maintain a healthy lifestyle all year round, except when they go on vacation. They're still careful, but during that one or two weeks of each year, they may enjoy an occasional indulgence. Maybe on a trip to an amusement park, they'll buy hot dogs, pop, even cotton candy. A day of sightseeing may include a stop for a burger and fries. Dinner may be finished with an indulgence from a dessert tray.

These people still take their vitamin and mineral supplements during vacation. They still do enough walking to count as adequate exercise. And they still make healthy choices from the full-service menus at their hotel restaurants. They've learned that moderation is critical.

Whatever your situation, remember that this is the diet you should follow while you are healthy. If you are diabetic, have heart disease, or another illness, then you do not have this flexibility. Appropriate food choices will make the difference between illness and wellness, between a rich, full life and the deterioration of your body. But if you're using this book as much to prevent a problem as to treat one, there's no reason you can't cheat occasionally.

So what should be in your basic diet to ensure natural healing? When you enter a supermarket, no matter how it's laid out, go to the produce section first. This is important, because if you're an impulse-buyer, the produce section is the safest place for you. Increasingly, large supermarket chains and health food stores are adding small sections of organically grown produce. If possible, always choose organic foods, because they are less likely to have been exposed to contaminants such as pesticides. Organic produce is not guaranteed to be pesticide-free, because no matter how careful the grower, the soil may have been contaminated by others. It is, however, probably safer for you than "regular" vegetables. In addition, a number of larger cities have begun hosting farmers' markets two or three days a week. You'll often be able to buy fresher produce there than you'll find in the stores. And you can learn about the growing methods, and then buy the food that's safest for your family.

Select any and all vegetables that are in season. Try new things! Be sure to get garlic if you can use it in cooking. Look for Kyolic garlic, both in the supermarket and in health food stores, because it is preferable to regular garlic and won't cause problems for most of the people who react adversely to garlic.

As you shop, plan some of your meals. Think about ways to use the produce in salads, by itself, in juices, and every possible way. Remember that vegetable and fruit can be used with poultry and fish to enhance the taste. You might want to skim through a cookbook before you go or just think about ways to blend flavors while you study what is available.

Think about meatless dishes you'd enjoy eating. There are many meatless pasta dishes that are so delicious, even meat lovers are surprised to find that they don't contain meat. More food stores now sell soy equivalents of meat products. Some hamburger substitutes have the taste of beef. There are meatless "meats" and combination products, like the croquettes I mentioned earlier.

Once you've done your exploring and selecting, look in the section that has rice, beans, and packaged soups. Avoid canned soups, which frequently have ingredients or additives that make them less nutritionally valuable than they seem. You can easily, of course, make your own nutritional soup with packaged beans and other mixes to which you add cut-up vegetables, maybe some meat (go easy), fowl, or fish.

If you like to snack, think about snacks you can make with cut fruit and vegetables. You can carry them in your purse or briefcase in a sealed plastic bag or other container.

A juicer is an ideal utensil to have in your kitchen; you can make fresh fruit and vegetable beverages. A useful juicer is likely to cost you no more than $150, an excellent investment. (Top-of-the-line juicers for home use can cost as much as $500, but they aren't necessary.) Then buy fresh fruits and vegetables and make them into juice. Many new canned and bottled beverages are quite healthy as well, but since the fresher the juice is, the better, it's good to have a juicer on hand.

If you're interested in cookbooks, look through the ones published for vegetarians, for those seeking low-fat meals, and for diabetics. Scan several to see which ones have recipes you know you'll enjoy. Also check those which feature Mediterranean-style cooking. Their heavy use of tomatoes, garlic (substitute Kyolic garlic), vegetable oils, and fish greatly reduce the risk of a variety of ailments. You can forgo the cost of many supplements and gain lots of the nutrients for which you've been taking capsules, tablets, powders, and liquids. And unlike supplements, the Mediterranean diet tastes delicious.

But the most important thing to remember is that there is no single way to fix a healthy meal. One person using one cookbook may produce bland, boring, almost tasteless food that makes healthy living seem a punishment. Another person, using a different cookbook, can produce gourmet meals that taste so good, you have to remind yourself that they're good for you, not indulgences. Take your time, and you'll find the books that work for you. Read through them when you're planning your meals.

Some of the other points to consider as you reconfigure your eating habits are really common sense. First, listen to your body. We usually know when we're eating the wrong foods, because our bodies tell us. We may joke about what we've done, but we're knowledgeable about our eating habits in the same way as we are about our body's health.

Weight maintenance follows a logical process. You achieve a constant weight when your body burns as many calories as it consumes. This doesn't mean that simply not gaining weight will keep you healthy. Even when your calorie intake and out-take are balanced, it does you little good unless you're balancing all the nutrients your body needs. I mean proteins, carbohydrates, and fats. And make sure you're getting all the essential vitamins and minerals.

Many of my patients are surprised to discover that when they eat foods with full nutritional value, they naturally have the right balance of fat and lean in their diets. They feel good; they don't gain weight, and they don't have to count their calories. They also tend not to overindulge because they're comfortable stopping when they've met their needs. Most of the people who overeat are those who lack the essential nutrients; they try to compensate by eating more inappropriate foods.

If possible, you might try eating four or five small meals a day. This will help your metabolism burn faster. If you take a brisk walk for twenty or thirty minutes before you eat, you'll also improve your metabolism. Getting your metabolism into a healthy balance is an excellent way to lose weight. Many diets suggest fasting—what amounts to starving your body—but that only triggers the body's defense mechanisms. Your body decides there's a famine in the land, and, determined to save your life, your body goes into a protective mode and begins to store fat. You're thinking weight loss. Your body is thinking biblically. It's acting as though the Lord has brought plagues and pestilence. That's why it's better for you to eat several small meals than to try to starve yourself.

Note: Fasting can be very important for the detoxification of the body. Periodic fasting, consuming juices for twenty-four hours but avoiding solid foods, can be important for your health. This is not meant to lose weight but to detoxify. While each person is different, I have found that fasting with juices— *not* a water only fast—one day a week and perhaps three or four days every three months is important for my health. For the longer fasts for detoxification, it is best to consult with a health care professional. In all cases, consume juices. The fast is solely from solid foods.

As for processed foods, remember that the processing has weakened their nutrients in a dangerous way. Essential vitamins and nutrients have been removed. You may eat your fill but not be in good health, because you lack what you need for the highest quality of life. You may age prematurely; perhaps die before your time. You'll certainly be less effective in what you try to do. This is why supplements are critical. This is why many of them can and will save your life.

3. *Rest.* You remember rest, don't you? It's that sixty-second period when you close your eyes and exhale while waiting at a traffic light during rush hour. It's those five minutes during which you go from typing on the computer to discovering your forehead bears the imprint of the keyboard, because you couldn't stay awake a moment longer. It's those three minutes and twenty-seven seconds of blessed silence between the time your child gets out of the car in front of his friend's house and the two of them come running to you to ask for a ride to the soccer game. It's that four- or five-hour time in bed, whether you need it or not, during which you sleep, think about what you didn't get done that day, or worry about what you have to do tomorrow. Some people do all three, of course, but as long as they're lying prone and their eyes are closed, they're resting.

Or is something wrong with this picture?

There are only two experiences in life when sleep deprivation is normal, expected, and beyond your ability to fix. One is when you're a prisoner of war on a forced march through enemy territory. The other is the first three to four months following the birth of each of your babies. Both lead to a certain amount of post-traumatic stress and the tendency to need to tell and retell the story of the experience.

Am I being facetious? Just a bit. In point of fact, we're a society that looks on rest as an enemy instead of the friend it is. We treat it as a disease to be avoided, in much the same way we avert our faces from colleagues with sniffling noses, watery eyes, and hacking coughs. We brag about how little sleep we get, how much we're accomplishing. But the truth is that many Americans are sleep-deprived, ensuring that their bodies are not functioning to their full ability.

For each and every one of us, rest is a time of healing. Rest is a time of recovery. Rest is a time of growth. Deprive a child of sleep, and he will not thrive. Over time, he'll be less resistant to disease, more susceptible to fears and worries.

Most of us have read with envy about the geniuses who brag that they accomplished all they did because they slept only four or five hours a night. This may be true in some instances, just as it's true that Albert Einstein required ten hours of sleep a night, two hours more than most of us consider ideal. What is not said is that few, if any, of those geniuses slept only the amount of time they said they did. For example, Thomas Alva Edison seldom spent more than four hours in bed, but what is not known so well is that he took catnaps throughout the day. His total sleep in a twenty-four-hour period isn't recorded, but it was surely closer to eight hours than to the four hours he actually spent in bed.

In recent months a number of sleep studies have found that individuals who nap for just twenty minutes during the course of a day are so refreshed that they're able to work with the same mental acuity as if they'd had a full night's sleep. The twenty-minute "jump start" is as useful for the person who came to work rested from a full night's sleep as it is for someone who tossed and turned all night.

Many businesses have failed to profit from this information, though some companies have paid heed. These companies encourage each employee to take a twenty-minute nap on company time, usually at some point after the lunch hour, when everyone is sluggish while metabolizing his food. They've found that those people who nap can perform as well during the afternoon as they did in the morning. Before the naps were permitted, afternoons were relatively unproductive times.

In another experiment, Irv Dardik, M.D., a research physician who has been head of sports medicine for the Olympic games, discovered that the resting cycle of an exercise program can be a time of healing. Using a special pulse-monitor watch, Dr. Dardik found a way to exercise to a predetermined maximum heart rate, then use relaxation and visualization techniques during the resting phase. He found that a person's health would improve and healing take place faster than normal if he took advantage of what most people think of as the "down-time" of exercise.

The point of all this is that sleep is a necessity for good health. That's why melatonin is important. That's why the successful person considers rest as vital as work.

Remember, what we're talking about is sleep, lying comfortably, with your eyes closed, in a dark room. We're not talking about relaxing with a good book, with music, with friends, or enjoying a hobby. Those are all pleasant and useful, but they do not provide the benefits of sleep.

The issue of rest quite apart from sleep is also important and is a related category. Many of us are unable to sleep unless we can relax from the cares of the day.

How do you relax and rest? Each of us does so in a different way. Some people use strenuous activity to relax, though they're really redirecting themselves into doing something that makes it easier for them to sleep.

For example, some people like to end their workday with a three- or four-mile walk. Sometimes they take the walk in the area where they work; perhaps they walk home, if it's a distance they can cover in no more than an hour. Sometimes they walk in the neighborhood where they live. Sometimes they walk in shopping malls, many of which encourage walkers. And sometimes they walk with a friend, lover, or pet.

Some people listen to music, though the kind of music they choose is critical. Music should quiet your body and your mind. It should help you relax, not make you excited.

If you're uncertain about what's best for you, try having breakfast and dinner in a coffee shop or restaurant where there's a music service like Muzak. The people who run such services are very careful to program their music the way you may program your day.

Listen to the music they choose to play in the morning. Often it is upbeat and fast-tempoed. Then, if you watch the people eating around you, you'll see that their movements seem almost choreographed to the music. We subconsciously react to tempo, to be hurried along by the right music.

Why? Because breakfast is a meal that usually has no side orders to add to our bill. If someone orders bacon, eggs, hash browns, toast, coffee, and juice, that's usually the final order. There won't be appetizers, additional drinks, or desserts. Therefore, the money the restaurant can earn is limited, and the best way to increase the take is to turn over the table. This means moving customers in and out quickly, replacing one set of diners with another. Fast, friendly service coupled with up-tempo music leads to the highest volume of business.

The evening is different. Most all-day restaurants have fewer customers for dinner than they do for breakfast. So instead of trying to move as many small orders as they can, they try to encourage the fewer customers to linger over more food, especially high-profit items.

Consequently, the music you'll hear will often be slower and more peaceful. The effect of this pleasant subconscious manipulation is that you may order drinks, whether liquor, soft drinks, or the fruit juices that are becoming popular in some upscale establishments. The server will be attentive, refilling your glass, perhaps letting you know that things are a little slow in the kitchen so maybe you'd like to have something more immediately. You'll probably order at least one appetizer, perhaps two drinks instead of one, and add a side order of soup or salad. You won't feel neglected, because the server is attentive, even if you're kept hungrier than is necessary for the real preparation time of your order. You may notice that the lights are dimmed to help your melatonin kick in, relaxing you. The music will be slow, gentle, the kind you might enjoy when lying on a couch, with your eyes closed.

Then, with the music still relaxing to listen to, you may be encouraged to have dessert and another drink. Each is a separate charge. Each adds to your bill. And because you've been lingering so peacefully, you find that you don't mind paying the high bill and a good tip. And most important, you're likely to return.

As music calms you in a restaurant, it brings you peace when you're unwinding from the day's activities. This is why I recommend using music to relax, selecting the type of restful pieces used by the programmer for the restaurant's dinner hour.

And there's nothing wrong with developing a hobby for relaxation, maybe taking up an absorbing sport, like tennis, martial arts, or ballroom or swing dancing. Maybe collecting stamps or dolls. The choice is yours. Whatever you do, though, you must separate the activity that is restful from true rest.

Sleep, critical for your health, is an essential component of all natural remedies. And just as you may have to shift your work schedule to address priorities on the job or with your family, so you may have to adjust your sleep schedule to ensure yourself adequate rest. If you can't get the proper amount of rest at night, then plan to take nap breaks. This is not time wasted. The proper amount of sleep will do more to help improve your performance than would the same amount of time spent on additional work or practice.

4. *Relationships.* People are not meant to live in isolation. We are rare among mammals in our ability to bond for a lifetime. What we often deny is that we need to bond, if not in marriage, then at least in friendships.

In recent years numerous studies have tried to determine what constitutes good emotional and physical health. One that I found especially interesting was carried out in Alameda County, California, by Lisa F. Berkman and Lester Breslow, published by Oxford University Press in 1983. They found that those who isolate themselves from the community have a greater risk of health problems than people who retain their sense of community. Their findings indicate that if you're in a close relationship, have friends in a religious group, club, or other close association, and have poor dietary and exercise habits, you may well be in better health and may live longer than a well-exercised "hard body" who has few, if any, close friends and who delights in being alone. This is true even if the first subject is a man who lives happily within a community but smokes, eats meat, and barely gets the proper amount of fresh fruit and vegetables, while the solitary person is careful about diet and supplements.

The Alameda project studied Japanese Americans in the area. They came from a long tradition of close community ties, and as long as they re-created these ties within their community in the United States, they had an unusually low rate of such stress-related ailments as cancer. And this was true even of those who smoked and had switched to a Western diet. By contrast, the Japanese who came to the United States and became thoroughly Westernized, and were comfortable living without the support of a strong community and extended family, saw their rate of stress-related illnesses drastically increase.

I've mentioned that early death was common among factory workers who retired. In the 1950s a large group of factory workers was studied in Detroit, Cleveland, Akron, and Pittsburgh. They were all in the same industry, manufacturing products used in automobiles. They all were under similar stress, earned similar pay, and had similar diets. Most drank alcohol, usually beer, and most smoked. Theoretically, then, they all should have died about the same age, but that turned out not to be true. The men who stayed home and lived isolated lives after retirement, even though they remained physically active around the house, were dead within three years. By contrast, men with the same health risks who joined clubs or became more active in the clubs to which they belonged, engaged in volunteer work, were involved in their religious communities, got part-time jobs, or otherwise found ways to interact with others, had much longer life spans—an additional ten to twenty years beyond that of their former co-workers who isolated themselves.

What this demonstrates is that people who are active in communities—and this can mean the family—seem to have a greater will to live. A man or woman experiencing a life-threatening illness or surgery has a better chance for recovery if she has a loved one—a spouse, a lover, an important close friend, or even a beloved pet. The will to live is triggered by the feelings nourished by close relationships. Being loved, being cared about, being a part of the group is the most healthful experience you can have.

Our need for community, even a community of two, is most evident when a troubled individual seeks counseling. The people of ancient times understood how important a caring listener can be. Some cities had paid listeners in the marketplace, men who, for a fee, listened to your troubles. They were compassionate, caring, understanding. We don't know whether they offered words of advice, though it's doubtful. Only later, when we developed fields like psychology and psychiatry, did the paid listener turn into a different kind of professional. Yet the health value was the same and remains so, whether the paid listener is a bartender, a member of the clergy, or a psychologist.

Loved ones perform this function, too. If we have the ability to talk through whatever is troubling us, we begin to heal.

Several years ago, two psychiatrists at the University of Washington School of Medicine in Seattle put together a scale that rated stress in a person's life. They worked out a point system for everything from the death of a spouse through divorce, marital separation, changing jobs, moving to a new city. If you wanted to work out your probability of health problems, all you had to do was list the significant changes you'd experienced in the previous twelve months, then add the corresponding points.

The Alameda study of Japanese Americans showed that this stress guide may not be as accurate as was originally thought. Suppose that a man in his seventies, living in New England, becomes widowed. Depressed, he decides he can't continue to live in the place where everything reminds him of what he had shared with the woman he loved. He packs his bags and moves to Arizona, where he knows no one but believes the climate will be pleasant. He rents an apartment, begins walking and watching his diet, and loses weight while becoming physically fit. He joins a church and participates in its activities. Several of the members become friends and call him daily, draw him into a social life, and nurture him through the first terrible year following his loss. Slowly, his health and his outlook on life improve.

Note: For most people, a church, synagogue, or mosque offers a convenient form of supportive community, which is why I mention them. Any group that provides such support, however, can work the same way. Some people join discussion groups. Other people join bowling leagues, where at least some of the members socialize outside the lanes. Still others join fraternal organizations or hobby clubs. What matters is person-to-person contact with caring people.

According to the point scale of the two psychiatrists, the man should be dead. But real life is something else. Certainly his immune system was under stress. The quality of his health was precarious. But in the embracing community, his immune system strengthened, his attitude became positive, and his health improved. Admittedly, he was at high risk for serious illness during the months after his wife died and he was still relocating. Some men and women don't survive the changes.

But when they do, it is participation in the community, and the knowledge that others genuinely care about them, that can swing the balance and improve their health.

Paul Horton, M.D., a psychiatrist and author of *Solace: The Missing Dimension in Psychiatry*, sees solace in the manner of comfort. Children who are frightened, lonely, or tired will often cling to a blanket, a favorite stuffed toy, or another object. Nighttime rituals may involve clutching this object, shifting to a particular position in bed, perhaps finding a special angle under the covers and on the pillow. Then, when they have this familiar feeling, angle, and loved object, they swiftly find peace and rest.

Teenagers are troubled by the lack of solace. Dr. Horton believes that their sense of alienation and their rebellion are connected with a search for solace. How do they get to this state? First, there is the natural separation from their parents. Then, there's the reality that most of them don't yet have close friends. Intimate companionship usually comes later, as most teens are too wrapped up in themselves or too worried about what their friends will think of them to reach out. They're ashamed to use the comforting objects of childhood, though it's not unusual to see a troubled teenager in bed clutching a favorite bear or other toy.

Dr. Horton feels that teens who play loud music or turn to drugs and alcohol are trying a new way to find solace as they work toward building relationships with friends and restructuring their relationships with their families.

For teens and adults, animals can provide some of the solace and health benefits. Alan Beck, Sc.D., and Aaron Katcher, M.D., report in their book *Between Pets and People* that one in five people with severe heart disease and no pets would die. The person who owned an enjoyable pet—a dog or a cat—or something less demanding, like a lovely goldfish in a bowl or aquarium, had a risk of dying that was three percent lower. This doesn't sound like a great difference, but when it's translated into the number of people who have severe heart disease, the figure of those whose lives are saved is thirty thousand each year.

As a religious man, I believe that it is important to build a relationship with God. I'm not certain that it matters how you establish this relationship with God. Each faith, maybe each religious group to which you belong, has its own beliefs, just as I have mine. One of them may be exactly the right way. I believe that a loving heart, a willingness to reach out, and a willingness to listen will help you establish that right relationship with the Lord. I believe that you and God make a community that can sustain you in times of unavoidable isolation.

Even if you are a person who does not believe, you must trust in relationships. We need one another, and when we share our lives in a meaningful way, the quality and, in many cases, the quantity of life we enjoy are greatly improved.

Many people widen their ability to find peace through meditation. They may practice one of any number of means for relaxation and inward calming—yoga, transcendental meditation, biofeedback, or fractional relaxation. It must, however, be part of a lifestyle that involves social interaction. Without the latter, the former will be far less effective in maintaining or improving your health.

Finally, and this may seem like a backlash against modern technology, get off the Internet and get a life!

The greatest danger to the emotional health of Americans is their growing reliance on computers for entertainment and social interaction. We play games on the computer, either from the CD-ROM drive or on the Internet. We explore personal interests on the Internet, from gardening to pornography. We join chat rooms and make cyber friends who care about us, care about our problems, are there when we're troubled. And many of these cyber friends genuinely are concerned, valuing the time they spend writing back and forth.

In our offices we send e-mail instead of leaving our cubicles and moving about, seeing others, sharing ideas. The e-mail is so much simpler, so much faster. In fact, many parents of college students find that they can get a response to an e-mail, but a letter is usually ignored.

And now there's the cyber café, a new kind of coffee shop. It may have computer terminals, outlets for you to plug in your notebook, or both. You can have coffee, doughnuts, and browse the Internet. In some cases, if you're attracted to another person in the café, you can arrange to exchange e-mail.

What a wonderful new world! So why aren't we having fun?

Studies show that heavy users of computers are likely to be depressed, and to have less healthy immune systems.

Part of the problem is the lack of bright, full-spectrum light. Late at night it's easy to enter the computer as womb, turning down the lights and working from the glow of the monitor. Even during the day we forget how light-deprived we are. By using the computer in a brightly illuminated room, ideally one with full-spectrum bulbs, you'll have greater emotional health. Since emotional health affects your immune system, this alone can help save your life. That, however, is only part of the problem.

A computer is not a friend; it can become a guarantor of a poor quality of life coupled with a shortened existence.

Human beings were made for physical interaction. The human voice can affect our body chemistry. The right voice, the right pitch and inflection, and we relax. Think of a singer who can deliver a ballad in a way that touches your heart. A good singer can make you cry, make you laugh, help you feel at peace.

The same thing happens when we have a conversation with another person. That's why lovers often say that they knew they'd found the right partner because they realized they'd been talking all night and felt wonderful.

Likewise the wrong voice—either of someone we dislike or words said in anger—can cause the fight-or-flight response. We get an adrenalin rush that will ultimately leave us hungry and exhausted. Over time, repeated experiences will weaken our immune system.

Human beings were made for touch. Holding someone we love leads to lower blood pressure, a slower heart rate, slower breathing, and a calmer, happier attitude. The same is true when we are touched.

There are questions being raised about touch therapy, a concept taught in a number of nursing schools. It is based on the idea that hands moving over an injured part of the body can lead to faster healing. A teenage girl arranged an experiment in which she found that moving hands over an infected part of the body did nothing to change healing. At the same time, many health professionals have found that therapeutic touching does speed recovery. Unfortunately, scientific studies have yet to be devised or reported.

What is not in question is that a loving, caring touch helps to strengthen the immune system. Many seriously ill people are—or think of themselves as—outcasts from society. Some have diseases like AIDS, which people fear and hold in disdain, because they think that contracting it speaks poorly for the person's moral character. Others have conditions that change their lives so drastically, they can no longer be a part of groups that previously served to validate their worth, at least in their own minds. Someone who has to retire from a management position because of a severe heart condition, for example, is suddenly left without human contact, without evaluation of her own work, without a way to validate her self-worth in ways that had become comfortable and familiar. Sometimes it is inconvenient to visit a person who is hospitalized, so the patient is alone. Whatever the reason, the isolation leads to depression that can be countered by hugs, touch, the physical attention that says she still matters.

Hospice workers understand this. All the people for whom they care are terminally ill, yet the workers hug them, touch them, stroke their brows, hold their hands, listen to what they have to say. And when the workers create such a relationship, the patient's quality of life is vastly improved, even if his death is still imminent. Consequently, when death occurs, that patient's end almost always comes more easily, as he has achieved emotional peace.

Our bodies do not need fantasy relationships. We do not need cyber friends, cyber sex, cyber guides. We need social interaction. We need real love, friends with whom we can physically interact, learning that enables us to spend time with faculty and classmates both in and out of sessions. There is great value to what is available through the Internet and other computer resources, but if the video monitor is your gateway to what you call friendship, your health is at risk.

5. *Supplements.* There is something frightening about going into a health food store for the first time. A well-stocked store has row after row of vitamin bottles, mineral bottles,

lotions, potions, organic foods, beverages . . . Th
seems endless, and to make matters worse, a well-stockea
store has price variations that make no sense. You pick up
a bottle of a hundred 1000-milligram vitamin C tablets
that is priced at twenty dollars, and then find the product
nearby for five dollars. Each is bottled by a different company. How do you choose?

You also realize, as you look around you and eavesdrop on
the other customers, that everything here has a purpose. It's all
good for you, all good for what ails you. (Or perhaps all good
for what *could* ail you that *wouldn't* ail you if you took the
product.) To say it's confusing is an understatement.

Adding to the confusion are physicians, and others concerned with natural therapies, who recommend a vitamin or
mineral supplement program involving so many different products that you begin to fear you may have a terminal illness.
Your day revolves around which vitamin or mineral to take and
when. You have supplements to take with breakfast, with
lunch, and with dinner. There are supplements to keep in your
pocket or purse, and supplements to store in your desk at work
in case of an unexpected bout of stress.

So what can you do? Take the supplements and use common sense.

First, take one multiple vitamin each day. Make certain it's
as complete as possible, containing both vitamins and minerals.
A good check is to see how large a dose you'll be getting of each
of the B-complex vitamins. The ideal is a multivitamin-mineral
tablet that has at least 50 milligrams or micrograms of each of
the B-complex vitamins. This is simple, not costly, and offers a
wide range of protection.

: garlic. All garlic is good for you if you can
ɡarlic is the ideal form for almost everyone
ntage of not causing a foul odor.

ɪsses mentioned earlier, especially barley green
ss. Check that chapter to see what to keep in
minɑ .   ju go to buy them.

You must have two antioxidants: vitamins C and E. The dose of each will vary according to the stress your body's under, but I recommend a minimum of 2000 to 5000 milligrams (2 to 5 grams) of vitamin C and between 400 IU and 1200 IU of vitamin E daily.

That broad range of vitamin E may seem strange, but at this point we still know little about it. Some studies recommend 400 IU as the minimum, and this seems convenient for many people. We also know, however, that men need more vitamin E than women do, and that the amount we need is related to body size. There are also studies indicating that a dose of 1200 IU of vitamin E is far too low. My personal choice is 800 IU to 1200 IU of vitamin E daily for everyone.

Next, you can boost the effectiveness of vitamins C and E by taking 200 micrograms a day of selenium, which may well be in your multiple vitamin. Also, try a newly understood substance called alpha lipoic acid (ALA). ALA and selenium conserve both vitamins C and E and allow them to fill their roles. Fifty to 250 milligrams per day is appropriate for ALA. I take the higher amount, but many studies indicate 50 milligrams is an effective minimum dosage.

The only other two supplements I recommend are (1) melatonin for everyone over forty, and (2) just for men over forty, something called lycopene. Lycopene is found in the red pigment of tomatoes and plays an important role in preventing prostate cancer. It cannot be destroyed by heating or cooling, so if you consume large quantities of tomato products, or if you drink two large glasses of tomato juice each day, you'll be obtaining it naturally.

Israeli agricultural scientists have developed a natural super tomato with five times more lycopene than your best garden-grown tomatoes. It is called Lycomato. An oleoresin extract of the Lycomato can be obtained in antioxidant and prostate support formulas. A daily intake of 5 to 10 milligrams is recommended.

AND IN CONCLUSION

I'd like to leave you with a simple, healthful message of the type my parents received and gave me when I was growing up. That is, I hope you'll eat right, drink plenty of liquids, get fresh air every day, and don't forget to enjoy a good night's sleep.

That advice is the cornerstone of good health as God intended. In an ideal community—one where good sense prevails over greed, naïveté, and the many other negatives we add to our lives and to our planet—you would not need more than that. You would not need this book. Unfortunately, I don't believe such communities exist. If they did, I'd move there and promote healthful living in that paradise.

The sad truth is that we've "blown it." We've been blessed with the brains and bodies to be stewards of the Earth. We know how to grow all the plants we need for health and how to identify which plants are natural medicines. We know how to divert water hundreds of miles from its natural pathway, as with Arizona's Colorado River Project, so we never again need to suffer drought or famine. We know how to care for livestock, how to improve soil, and how to ship meat and produce thousands of miles so that people can build settlements in barren areas. But instead of delighting in our abundance, we take much for granted and use the rest with greed.

In ignorance and arrogance we tossed toxic waste into the ocean, thinking the waters were so vast that the waste would disappear. We filled the sky with pollution, thinking its capacities were limitless, and we exhausted our food chain, thinking its resources were limitless. All of these excesses have led to the breakdown of a system more delicately balanced and interdependent than we realized.

At the moment, our planet appears potentially resilient. There is hope that the future will be better than the present, if we use our knowledge and abandon our greed. But, for the foreseeable future, certainly in my life and the lives of my loved ones, we also need to accept that my parents' generation's advice is now incomplete.

We all need the natural remedies discussed in this book. We all need the supplements and lifestyle modifications that will prevent many of the conditions mentioned in these pages. We all need to recognize that we have failed as stewards of Creation. Although it appears that we can redeem ourselves through change, that change will require at least two or three generations to become effective.

As a result, I leave you with the knowledge I have gained through my work as a doctor, a student of natural remedies, and a researcher into the work of others. Please write to me in care of the publisher to let me know how you're doing. I'm interested, and I care.

Appendix A

BECAUSE BIO-OXIDATION THERAPY has a great many concerns, the following additional information is of value.

The sources of information about ozone originally were published outside the United States. This is because most of the research and the use of these techniques have occurred in Europe and Russia, and more recently in Cuba. One of the standard early texts was the book *The Use of Ozone in Medicine* by Siegfried Rilling, M.D., and Renate Viebahn, M.D., Heidelberg: Haug Publishers, 1983. Over a thousand articles have been published in medical literature since the medical uses of ozone were taken seriously beginning in the 1930s. However, because the Medical Society for Ozone is located in Germany, Austria, Italy, and Switzerland, and because it works closely with the National Center for Scientific Research in Cuba, the German language, and to a lesser degree Russian and Spanish, have been the original languages of the papers. Only as they have been translated into English have Americans and Canadians been aware of the work. While U.S. physicians are behind in all this despite a body of evidence of success that is now leading to serious research and a clamoring for some treatments, most papers remain the domain of non–U.S. writers (e.g., *The Canadian Medical Association Journal* article by A. C. Baggs, M.D.—"Are Worry-Free Transfusions Just a Whiff of Ozone Away?" [April 1, 1993]). There have also been articles by

Americans looking at the experiences of doctors in other countries, such as the American *Journal of Public Health Policy*, Vol. 12, No. 1 (Spring 1991), in which writer Margaret Gilpin wrote "Update-Cuba: On the Road to a Family Medicine Nation."

Intra-Muscular Injection: Currently this procedure is most commonly used in Europe. It is a popular treatment for allergies and inflammatory diseases such as arthritis. It is also sometimes used as an adjunct to more traditional cancer therapies (though *not* as a substitute for traditional treatments).

Rectal Insufflation: A German surgeon, Dr. Erwin Payr, and a French physician, Dr. P. Aubourg, are considered the first users of rectal insufflation to treat medical problems. The two men used ozone gas in this manner for the treatment of mucous colitis and fistulae. This was in the 1930s. A decade later Dr. Payr began injecting ozone intravenously to treat circulatory disturbances. Today it is most commonly used in Cuba, Germany, and Russia. Some Americans with cancer and other diseases related to the immune system have tried self-treating themselves in this manner.

Ozone Bagging: Dr. Gerard V. Sunnen has reported on this and other procedures in the fall 1988 *Journal of Advancement in Medicine*, No. 3, in an article entitled "Ozone in Medicine: Overview and Future Direction." Dr. Sunnen found that when the skin absorbs the ozone, it is able to penetrate the capillaries enough to raise blood oxygen pressure. This is believed to influence the body's biochemistry.

Fractionalization: A number of European physicians delight in this treatment, technically known as autohomologous immunotherapy, or AHIT. It has not been around very long, having been developed in the 1980s by a German, Dr. Horst Kief, and it has not been approved for use in the United States. The European uses have shown no reported adverse side effects of which

I am aware. It is most commonly used for chronic infections, bronchial asthma, rheumatic joint diseases, and even cancer. Its use in the treating of cirrhosis, HIV-related illnesses, and other concerns is being studied. The major source of information comes from Horst Kief himself in the monograph *The Auto-homologous Immune Therapy* (Ludwigshafen: Kief Clinic, 1992).

Ozone and Oil: This is quite safe because it is applied as a salve or balm. It is a procedure developed in Cuba for the treatment of a wide range of skin and fungal disorders, including bedsores, herpes simplex, insect bites, athlete's foot, leg ulcers, acne, and other, similar problems.

Intra-Articular Injection: Once again this is a therapy most common to the three countries long interested in the use of ozone for medical purposes—Germany, Cuba, and Russia. It is a common treatment for joint diseases such as arthritis. Ozone gas is bubbled through water, then injected directly into the joints.

Ozonated Water: This is a simple idea some dentists have used as a disinfectant during some oral surgeries. The ozone gas is allowed to bubble up through the water and the resultant liquid is used as a bath. In addition to its dental application, it has been used to cleanse some wounds and skin infections.

Russian physicians have used sterilized ozonated water as an irrigant during surgeries. And both Russian and Cuban physicians have experimented with its use for ulcers, diarrhea, ulcerative colitis, and similar intestinal problems. Dr. Gerard Sunnen has introduced this information to American doctors through his writing, but at this time it is not in use.

Autohemotherapy: This is the most common ozone therapy in the world. A combination of ozone and oxygen is bubbled through a quantity of blood taken from the patient, then the ozone/oxygenated blood is returned to the patient. Major autohemotherapy involves the removal of between 50 and 100 milliliters of blood for the treatment, after which it is returned through a vein. Minor autohemotherapy requires the removal of usually no more than 10 milliliters of blood, which is returned through intramuscular injection. The idea is to use the patient's own body chemistry to create a self-vaccine.

Currently this type of treatment is being used in Cuba in conjunction with the treatment of arthritis, cancer, heart disease, herpes, and HIV infection. In other countries, such as Russia, physicians use it to treat a broad range of health problems. It is safe enough that a search of the literature has not revealed problems.

THE DANGEROUS REMEDIES

Physicians regularly argue over the value of international medical research. Different countries have different standards for testing. Some are at least as thorough as those in the United States both in their research into pharmaceuticals before they are introduced on the market and in their development of treatment procedures for various ailments. For years there was a scandal looming over critically needed medicines that had been tested in countries with standards as high as or higher than those in the United States which could not be used here until another seven years of testing, on average, had taken place. Now many changes are occurring, some made more urgent because of epidemics such as HIV. At the same time, the use of the Internet has allowed desperately ill individuals as well as individuals who don't trust contemporary medicine no matter how successful it has proven to be to discover a wealth of medical information. Unfortunately at least some of that information is outdated and potentially dangerous.

The procedures listed under the dangerous therapies section—injection into veins or arteries and ozone inhalation—are known in literature readily available on the Internet and elsewhere. What is not so commonly known is that they have been used enough for physicians to realize that they cannot be controlled in an effective manner. Even the most skilled physician is likely to have an unacceptable error rate with their use. They are mentioned here because you may have read about them elsewhere. They are not mentioned as something to be sought out. Already physicians in the countries where they have been utilized—countries such as Russia, Germany, Cuba, and the like—are abandoning them. And these are the countries with the longest history of both experimentation and successful utilization.

Index

James F. Balch, M.D., is the coauthor of the bestseller *Prescription for Nutritional Healing* and the author of other alternative health books, including *The Super Antioxidants*. For more than thirty-five years he has been a medical doctor and surgeon who, twenty years ago, began to see the life-changing benefits of alternative medicine not taught in medical school. Today he writes books and is a world lecturer, teaching the incredible benefits of alternative health styles.

Printed in the United States
17940LVS00002B/109-114

9 780385 493505